WHEN CARING
TAKES COURAGE

Alzheimer's/Dementia:
At-a-Glance Guide for Family Caregivers

2ND EDITION

Mara Botonis

outskirtspress
DENVER, COLORADO

Dedication

This book is dedicated to the memory of my beloved grandfather, Bill.

Thank you for the example you provided for all of us.

You are forever the standard by which I measure myself.

Foreword

I recall as a 21 year-old being asked by the administrator of the nursing home where I held a summer job to run a group treatment program for residents suffering Alzheimer's Dementia (AD). The hope was that we could help reduce loneliness and symptoms of depression for the residents who participated. During my work at the nursing home, I learned about the significant variability of behavior demonstrated by persons suffering AD. I also learned how hard and how intimidating it is to care for someone with a progressive dementia.

Thirty years later I have had the distinct pleasure of caring for hundreds of persons suffering AD and related dementias. I have seen firsthand the extraordinary emotional and financial distress AD can place on the family caregivers. Such situations also teach us about the greatness of the human spirit and the power of love. Thirty years later I am *reminded* how hard and how intimidating it is to care for someone with a progressive dementia.

Serving the role of caregiver is something most of us are not prepared for. There are over 15 million caregivers of those with AD in the United States and this number will more than double by the middle of this century. Nearly 30% of these caregivers will experience symptoms of clinical depression and more will suffer high levels of stress. Unfortunately, nearly 100% of caregivers are not prepared for caring for someone with a progressive dementia. It is not the type of learning or information we seek in our daily lives. Caregivers therefore can feel lost, afraid, guilty, and frustrated as they deal daily with a disease process that is difficult to understand.

Mara Botonis has written this wonderful book, When Caring Takes Courage, which provides caregivers with a practical guide for interacting and caring for their loved one with dementia. In so doing, Mara has provided everyone with an "at-a-glance" resource and "go-to" guide. In this book, readers will glean practical tips from family caregivers, learn effective methods for how to provide care from healthcare professionals, and obtain over 700 Alzheimer's adapted activity ideas that they can try at home. Most importantly, Mara's book helps to reduce the uncertainty, guilt, fear, and intimidation of being a caregiver.

Each of the chapters are easy to read and filled with meaningful tips. Throughout the book, readers will find many interactive tools that they can personalize to help them with planning and providing important elements of their loved ones care. *Congratulations to Mara Maitlin Botonis for writing this <u>need to read guide</u> for all current and future caregivers in our nation.*

Her information is not developed from a clinical or academic perspective. Rather, the text is born from a personal and most meaningful experience of learning many families cope when a loved one is stricken with Alzheimer's/dementia. Mara was extremely close to her grandfather. His struggle and eventual death from this disease not only fueled in part the writing of this needed guide, it served as an important factor for her professional work within the senior housing and senior care industry.

I can enthusiastically recommend this text to all those who are now in the noble and loving role of caregiver. I also encourage the millions of people who are not yet serving in the role of caregiver to read this book to become educated and prepared for a future time when you may be needed.

Paul D. Nussbaum, Ph.D., ABPP
Brain Health Center, Inc.
Clinical Neuropsychologist
United Nations Presenter: Brain Health
Co-Founder, Chief Science Officer for Fit Brains
www.brainhealthctr.com
www.paulnussbaum.com

Mara Botonis

After thirty years in healthcare, working throughout the United States in the senior housing industry, Mara's life and career trajectory was forever changed when a close family member was stricken with Alzheimer's. When the Grandfather that served as her primary paternal influence for over 40 years began losing access to the memories that made up his life story, she knew she had to do something to help. Her everyday work at the national level alongside family care partners as well as countless medical and healthcare professionals offered unparalleled opportunities to learn from their collective expertise.

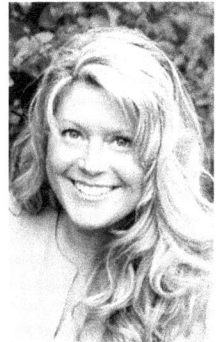

Mara called in all of her favors and spent five years researching and working on her-at-a-glance care guide; "When Caring Takes Courage". Her self-published book was produced with her husband's support using their life savings and contains over 1,000 quick tips for other family caregivers, compiled in a way that is practical and user friendly. Mara continues to be an active volunteer and in-demand speaker for healthcare professionals and family caregivers.

Volunteer roles have included:
Alzheimer's Association-Chapter Board Member
National Dementia Action Alliance-Access and Utilization Co-Chair
Project Lifesaver International-Law Enforcement Alzheimer's Educator
US Against Alzheimer's-National Support Group Co-Moderator
Caregivers.com-Web Content Curator

Contributing writer for:

Alzheimer's Foundation of America's *Care Quarterly*
www.about.com
www.alz.live
www.alzheimers.net
www.alzheimersreadingroom.com
www.aplaceformom.com
www.commonsensecaregiving.com
www.huffintonpost.com
www.senioradvisor.com
www.seniorcare.com
www.mariashriver.com

Recognized As:

Best -Selling Author, "When Caring Takes Courage"
2015 Recipient of the Jefferson Award for Outstanding Public Service
2015 National Jacqueline Kennedy Onassis Medal Honoree-Outstanding Public Service
2015 Treasure Coast Healthcare Champion Finalist
Maria Shriver's Architect of Change, Women's Alzheimer's Challenge

Acknowledgments

First and foremost, I want to thank my husband, **Dr. David Botonis**. He is my most meaningful mentor, my best friend, my love and my life. He is the reason you are reading this book, because without him, it would not have been possible. I love you, Honey. Forever and always.

Thank you to my amazingly selfless and noble Mom, **Cathy**. Your daily sacrifices for your children and your parents taught me what unconditional love really is. Your influence and guidance is felt on every page of this book and I am forever grateful for all of the loving care you put into helping other family caregivers coping with the effects of Alzheimer's. "I loved you first".

To **Paul Nussbaum, Ph.D., ABPP** who's tireless efforts and research into brain health have created new hope around the idea that it is never too late to improve your quality of life and over all well-being. Thank you for teaching us to better appreciate the remarkable gifts and possibilities that exist in our own minds. You have taught and inspired a countless number of healthcare providers, brain enthusiasts of all ages and created new hope around the idea that our brain can improve, can continue to learn and grow at any age. I admire you with my whole hippocampus! Learn more about his important work and your own brain health at: www.paulnussbaum.com.

I am eternally grateful to **Naomi Feil, M.S.W., A.C.S.W.,** pioneer of Validation Therapy which forever changed the landscape of caregiving for persons with Alzheimer's and Dementia. It is because of her we no longer feel the need to constantly "correct and re-direct" our loved ones and instead can connect based on what they are feeling. Her work and mission are located on the site: htttps://vfvalidation.org.

Thank you to **Lori La Bey**, of Alzheimer's Speaks, Dr. Oz's #1 Online Alzheimer's Influencer (https://www.alzheimersspeaks.com/) for the ego-less way she seeks to unite and give voice to every person impacted by dementia. For over 30 years, Lori learned firsthand by caring for her mother how to help Dorothy live well with dementia in spite of the disease.

With the curiosity of a family caregiver and the perspective of a global dementia advocate, Lori expertly brings worldwide dementia care innovators into our homes every week through her program "Alzheimer's Speaks Radio" for "kitchen table" style conversations that makes new information and ideas easy to digest for anyone dealing with the impact of dementia and are available on demand whenever we have a few minutes in our hectic schedules to take a listen. Whether you are a professional provider, informal family caregiver, person living with dementia or someone who hadn't heard of Alzheimer's until you watched the Oscar nominated film, "Still Alice", Lori has a way of inviting you into the conversation with the warmth of a friend and then challenging you to be a part of the solution with the familiarity of an elder sibling. Her "Oprah-esque" style at once re-affirms the value of your voice and your personal experience and then encourages a greater sense of personal responsibility in using that power collectively to positively impact the greater good. Thank you for being a daily inspiration and dear friend.

To the residents, staff, and volunteers at various Senior Living providers from whom I learned a great deal about Alzheimer's and Dementia over the past 30+ years in the healthcare industry.

To the leadership and volunteers of the outstanding Alzheimer's advocacy organizations I had had the privilege of serving alongside; the **Alzheimer's Association,** the **Alzheimer's Foundation of America**, the **National Dementia Action Alliance**, **UsAgainstAlzheimer's** and **Project Lifesaver International**.

And finally and most importantly, to the thousands of family caregivers I have had the privilege of talking with over all of those years. Your courage and grace, which are often unsung and unnoticed, are nothing short of heroic. You are amazing, you are doing the right things, and every single time you get through another day, you are successful.

Thank you for the nights you didn't get any sleep because you needed to be ever vigilant, for the times your meal was cold when you finally got to eat it, for the way you would steel yourself against harsh words and false accusations from the very person you were trying to help. Thank you for enduring the pain that comes with the loss of recognition and coping with the grief that comes from taking care of someone you cherish when they don't even know who you are or where they are. Thank you for all the times you make sure clean clothes are ready, food is prepared, dishes are done, housework is caught up, medications are given, bathing is accomplished, appointments and transportation have been coordinated, bills and mail are handled, toileting reminders and "accidents" are handled and all of the other countless daily tasks that fall on your shoulders are completed.

Thank you for all the times you feel like your whole world, your whole life is given in service to your loved one. For the vacations you didn't get to take, the days off you don't ever seem to get anymore, the "having a moment to yourself" that has become a distant memory, for all the days when you feel like you can't even take time to get your own shower, for the television shows and movies you've skipped, for the pleasure reading you can't seem to find time for, the friends you have missed, the outings to places other than doctor's offices, grocery stores and pharmacies that are now a thing of the past, for the hobbies you used to enjoy but have no time for. Thank you for being who you are, for setting aside big parts of own needs to give more to someone else. Thank you for answering the call. Thank you for rising to the need every moment, every hour, every day, and every time. For getting up each day and doing it all over again, even when you are exhausted, when you are sad, when you are sick, when you are lonely, when you are frustrated, when you are confused and when you feel all alone. You are not!

Thank you to all of these sons, daughters, wives, husbands, grandchildren, siblings and families and medical professionals who care for someone with Alzheimer's or Dementia. Thank you for helping me to share this empowering message with other family caregivers. Thank you for encouraging other caregivers to hang in there just a little while longer. Thank you for showing that a better, brighter day is still ALWAYS possible.

Preface

"It's an honor and a privilege." Those are the words I shared with my mother during a phone call when I learned that she and my step-dad were moving in with my grandparents and would help to care for my grandfather, who was just starting to show signs of Alzheimer's.

During that talk, several years ago, so many thoughts were racing through my mind. How much more quality time would we have with my grandfather? When would he start to forget us, forget his wife of 60+ years? How lucky for my grandparents that their daughter, my mom was able to move in with them and help care for them in their home despite the increased care needs that the future would bring to delay the need for placement in an Alzheimer's community or hiring of professional caregivers. I remember thinking, how could this be happening to Grandpa? To us?

Looking back, I see that at the moment of that call, not only were our lives as a family forever changed but it also completely altered the trajectory of my life and career. I had worked with seniors as a direct caregiver during college and then moved into administration and marketing in the senior housing industry for over 29 years.

Helping seniors had been my passionate purpose since I was 14 and got my parents' permission to volunteer in a nursing home in upstate New York on summer vacation, not because I needed to but because I wanted to. Not many 14-year-olds on break choose to spend their time emptying bedpans and changing soiled linens just to have a few moments each day to connect with elderly patients they barely knew, but I did. And I loved getting to know them, getting to learn their life stories.

My journey evolved into marketing positions when an administrator saw me give a weekend tour to a family at the assisted living facility. It became my job to listen and learn from every family who inquired, and identify what was most important to them in choosing the right community for placement and then move their loved one in as quickly as possible so that they could get the help they needed. A string of accomplishments followed: national awards for high occupancy and record-setting new admission numbers, customer service, and customer feedback recognition awards, and promotion after promotion taking me up through the ranks from area, to regional, to divisional and then eventually to national director of sales and marketing-memory care for one of the country's largest providers of assisted living.

But from the moment my mother and grandmother shared with me my grandfather's diagnosis, everything changed. Though my role at work was still the same, my motivation was completely different. I read every Alzheimer's related article I could get my hands on; I learned everything I could from every nurse and neurologist and Alzheimer's organization I encountered nationwide. I gleaned everything I could from every family story I heard or read about across the country during my role as national director of marketing-memory care. These 100's and 100's of families, through their stories of real struggle, genuine hope and even happiness living with Alzheimer's and dementia became my mentors. I began to learn what worked best for caregivers at home. I discovered how to handle difficult behaviors and manage caregiver burnout. I was exposed to new ideas about how to carve out space for joy, how to live with the sadness and mitigate the guilt. Most importantly, I was learning how to do everything possible to prolong the amount of quality time families could have with their loved ones at home. In short, I was learning without realizing it, how to do the opposite of what my job required, I was learning how to help families impacted by Alzheimer's/dementia keep their loved one safely at home as long as possible. I learned how to help caregivers have the greatest number of the best possible days together for as long as possible. I was learning how to help my grandfather by helping the women who loved and cared for him at home. I was learning in a way that very few others before me have. I was learning firsthand from one of the biggest pools of family caregivers and Alzheimer's professionals across the country what success looks like for families coping with this disease.

It would be ten more years before I would be at a place and time in my life when I would finally get the chance to compile and share that information here with you.

According to the Alzheimer's Association (www.alz.org), "There are currently 5.3 million Americans living with Alzheimer's disease. By 2025, that figure will increase 40% to 7.1 million Americans. By 2050, without a medical breakthrough to slow or prevent the disease, that figure will triple over today's numbers and affect up to 16 million Americans." Currently, a whopping 80 percent of those living with Alzheimer's are cared for at home by a family member. That means there are over 15 million family caregivers striving to cope with the new and difficult challenges that caring for a loved one with this disease bring on a daily basis.

This book was lovingly written in honor of these family caregivers whose noble sacrifices often go unnoticed and unappreciated. On the following pages is a guide intended to accompany the family caregiver while navigating the unpredictable and unique path that this disease thrusts upon them. It contains best practices, tried and true solutions, step by steps "how-to's" and things to consider. It is designed to offer caregivers the information they need to make the best possible choices for their loved ones and themselves. This book represents the best advice I could find from persons living with dementia, neurologists, doctors, nurses, care aides, memory care program directors, wives, husbands, sons and daughters, grandchildren and friends around the country that are proving every single day that there can still be joy and hope and even happiness in a life touched by Alzheimer's disease.

I would also like to acknowledge the following leaders in dementia (including Alzheimer's) advocacy for their example and inspiration. Your work forever changed the face of healthcare. It was an honor to have the opportunity to work, volunteer, talk with and learn from you.

Alzheimer's Association
Alzheimer's Foundation of America
A Place for Mom
Amelia Wilson

Alzheimer's Reading Room
Bob DeMarco
Alzheimer's Speaks
Lori La Bey

Alz.Live
Dave Kelso
Autumn Leaves
Anna Forster, CPD
Best Friends Approach
Virginia Bell, MSW
David Troxel
Brain Health Center
Paul Nussbaum, Ph.D., ABPP
Brookdale (Emeritus) Senior Living:
Adora Brouillard
John Cincotta
Glenda Coots
Melissa Bean Day
Beth Dutton
Christopher Guay
Christopher Hyatt
Wendy McKenna, RN, BSN
Megan Pletcher
Crystal Roberts
Steve Sacco
Jayne Sallerson
Kelly Scott
Donald C. Tawney
Damon Thomas
April Harvoth Young
Care Changers
Michael Neuvirth
Cascade Living Group
Debbie Walker, RN
Cognitive Dynamics
Daniel C. Potts, MD, FAAN
Ellen Woodward Potts

Common Sense Caregiving
Gary Joseph LeBlanc
Creating Moments of Joy
Jolene Brackey
Dementia Action Alliance
Ellen Belk
Jayne Clairmont
Walter Coffey
Michael Ellenbogen
Michele Laughman
Karen Love
Kim McRae
Lori Smetanka
Louise Ryan
MaryAnn Sterling
Jackie Pinkowitz
Dementia Mentors
Truthful Kindness
Harry Urban
Karen Francis, MSW, CDP
Enlivant Senior Living
Tiffany Gentry Cobern Glatz
Evergreen Health
Kendra DeYoung Gunhold, MSW
Heavenly Care
Alice Latino
Seniorliving.net
Deborah Graves Collar
Help Stamp OUT Alzheimer's
Lynda Everman
Kathy Siggins
Hospice of Arizona
Annella Ritter

JEA Senior Living:
Alisa Anderson-Clark
Sue Johnston
Tod Murray
Rena Martinez Phillips
Kathleen Price
Learning to Speak Alzheimer's
Joanne Koenig Coste
Living Care Senior Housing
Delia McGinnis
Living Well with Alzheimer's
Dr. David Kramer
Memory People
Rick Phelps
Leeanne Chames
Meridian Senior Living:
Peter "Kacy" Kang
Robert Arsenault
Kevin Carlin
Kayla Wersel
National Health Investors
Justin Hutchens
Positive Approach Care (PAC)
Robin Andrews
Teepa Snow
Project Lifesaver International
Chief Tommy Carter
Crystal Gonzales
Elizabeth Kappes
Joe Salenetri
Chief Gene Saunders
Jeanne O'Neal Saunders

Sodalis Elder Living
Mark Rushing
SUNY Empire State College:
Theresa Maher
Sutter Coast Hospital
Beth Dalzell Liles
The Long and Winding Road
Ann Napoletan
Third Age Services
Carol Larkin, MA, CMC, CAEd, QDCS, EICS
USAgainstAlzheimer's
Carol Bradley Bursack
Virginia Bigger
Jessy Price Parrot
Sally Sacher
Loretta Woodward Veney
George Vradenburg
Trish Vradenburg
Validation Institute:
Naomi Feil, M.S.W., A.C.S.W.
Healthcare Retirees/Alumni
Alexander "Sandy" Halperin
A. Ellen Harris
Lynelle Lawson
Dawn Marsh
Suzette McCanliss
Kenny Pulsifer
Susan Scherr
Tony Walker
Elisa VanWinkle Wilson
In Memorium:
Patricia "Trish" Miller
Richard Taylor

Using this Book

This book is intended to be a quick, "go-to" reference for family caregivers. Reading it cover to cover or in sequential order is not necessary. Choose the chapters that best answer current questions or challenges and read the rest when you have the time or when the need arises. In my conversations with many families over the years, the common complaint I heard about existing books was that they were either way too detailed or that they simply did not have the time to read a lengthy book. This handbook is about helping you in those moments when Dad won't put on his pants or refuses to take his medication, for when Mom refuses to bathe, or you are having trouble getting your wife in the car to go to the doctor's appointment. This book is designed to help you reach your loved one again and reconnect when they may spend a big part of their day feeling lost or withdrawn. Hopefully, this book will help you to find more smiles and less stress in your day and to have at your finger-tips an at-a-glance guide to help you survive and thrive no matter what's happening at home.

My hope is that you think of this manual like your favorite cookbook. Please "dog ear" the pages that helped, scribble notes all over, skip parts you may not need right now and mix in your own recipe for successful caregiving along the way adding and subtracting from the best practices on these pages to assemble something that works best for you and your loved one.

You may not want or be ready for all of the information that is in this book right now, but I want you to have as much information as possible before you need it.

DISCLAIMER: *This book is intended as a general reference and in no way makes any specific guarantees or promises regarding outcomes or experiences using the techniques* *or ideas expressed in this book. Ideas contained herein are subject to specific approval by your family's personal physician before implementation. You should also seek medical advice before starting new caregiving approaches or techniques.*

Contents

SECTION TWO: COPING STRATEGIES FOR CARE PARTNERS

APPENDIX

SECTION ONE:
Helping Our Loved Ones Live Well

CHAPTER 1

Alzheimer's and Dementia – Signs and Symptoms for Family Self-Assessment

Alzheimer's is a type of dementia (the most common type) that causes problems with a person's memory, thinking and behavior. Dementia is an umbrella term describing the symptoms of many diseases and disease processes. Dementia itself is not a specific disease, but a cluster of symptoms such as personality changes, the inability to perform routine tasks, severe memory loss, and confusion. Many diseases and maladies can cause Dementia – some of those diseases are reversible and some are not. According to the Alzheimer's Association (www.alz.org), "Alzheimer's is not the only cause of memory loss. Many people have trouble with memory loss — this does not mean they have Alzheimer's. If you think your loved one may be exhibiting signs and symptoms of Dementia, which are not a normal part of aging, you should contact your medical provider right away." One of the things your medical providers may try to do initially is rule out any reversible causes of Dementia such as reaction to medications, urinary tract or other infection, dehydration, malnutrition, acute illness and depression to name a few.

The Alzheimer's Association notes that "Alzheimer's worsens over time and becomes progressively debilitating eventually causing the loss of both cognitive and physical functions. In its early stages, memory loss can be mild, but with late-stage Alzheimer's, individuals lose the ability to communicate; refuse to eat or forget to swallow; lose control of bowel and bladder; forget how to walk; sleep more and are unable to respond to their environment, often needing total assistance for all activities."

Our brains, like the rest of our bodies, change with age. Eventually, most of us notice a bit of slowed thinking and even occasional problems with remembering certain things. However, with Alzheimer's, serious memory loss, confusion and other major changes in how our minds work can be a signal that brain cells are failing in a way that is not typical in normal aging.

The Alzheimer's Association goes on to note that "the most common early symptom of Alzheimer's is difficulty remembering newly-learned information because Alzheimer's changes typically begin in the part of the brain that affects learning. As Alzheimer's advances through the brain, it leads to increasingly severe symptoms, including disorientation, mood, and behavioral changes; deepening confusion about events, time, and place; unfounded suspicions about family, friends and professional caregivers; more serious memory loss and behavior changes, and difficulty speaking, swallowing and walking."

According to the Alzheimer's Association's most recent "Facts and Figures Report" (available on their website at www.alz.org), "Alzheimer's is currently the sixth leading cause of death in the United States. Currently, Alzheimer's has no known cure, but there are some treatments available that may help slow the progression of symptoms and research continues."

The Alzheimer's Foundation of America (www.alzfdn.org) reports that according to recent research, "Alzheimer's disease typically progress over two to twenty years, and individuals live on average for eight to ten years from diagnosis. Individuals with Alzheimer's disease are likely to develop co-existing illnesses and most commonly die from pneumonia."

However, current treatments may temporarily slow the worsening of Dementia symptoms and may improve the quality of life for those with Alzheimer's and their caregivers. Today, there is a global effort underway to find better avenues to not only diagnose and treat the disease, but also to delay its' onset, and possibly prevent it from developing. New studies and findings are being frequently announced, so endeavor to keep abreast of the latest developments (see a directory of Alzheimer's websites and organizations in the Appendix).

This information may be demoralizing, and it's sad to acknowledge that each day you are fighting a disease that has no current cure, but remember, even though we can't change the destination, we can certainly alter the journey. This book is about empowering you to create the best possible day for you and your loved one in spite of this disease. No matter how much time you have left to spend with each other or what that time together may look like, we want you to have multiple resources at your fingertips to support you in enjoying those days as much as possible.

Persons with memory loss or other possible signs of dementia (including Alzheimer's) may find it hard to recognize or admit that they have a problem. Signs of dementia may be more obvious to family members or friends. If you feel that your loved one is experiencing Dementia-like symptoms, they should see a doctor as soon as possible.

Your local Alzheimer's Association chapter can help you find a physician who has experience diagnosing and treating memory problems. Early diagnosis, treatment, and intervention methods are improving dramatically and can greatly enhance the quality of life. If your loved one already has a preliminary diagnosis, it is still very important that you communicate the right kind of information to your physician about what you see at home so effective treatment options can be discussed and changed as needed along the way.

For more information about Alzheimer's disease and related dementias contact:

- **The Alzheimer's Association**: Website: www.alz.org or call their 24-hour helpline: 800-272-3900.

- **The Alzheimer's Foundation of America**: Website: www.alzfdb.org or call 866-232-8484 to be connected to their licensed social workers.

Let's take a closer look at what some of the most common symptoms look like:

☐ Severe Memory Loss: Repetitive questions, problems remembering names of people, places or things, unable to recognize their own children or grandchildren. Cannot state address, name next of kin. May resort to describing things they can no longer name, or seem to have "word salad" (right words in the wrong order when speaking or using the wrong word altogether).

☐ Confusion or Loss of Reasoning: No longer able to problem-solve, cannot understand "why." Cannot understand explanations, unable to apply logic to weigh consequences and choices. This leads to poor judgment such as dressing inappropriately for the weather, crossing dangerous streets, trusting strangers or taking things they like without realizing the item belongs to someone else.

☐ Personality Changes: Poor control over emotions, a response not commensurate with stimuli, easily frustrated, quicker to anger, lack of filter i.e. your loved one may say or do things that they never would've said before the disease, unable to follow social "norms." May appear withdrawn or remote.

☐ Inability to Perform Routine Tasks: Getting dressed, finding their way home after a short walk, writing their full name, tasks that require sequential steps done in a certain order become difficult. Inability to follow complex directions verbally, reading comprehension deteriorates, ability to process information visually is also impacted.

Symptoms of Alzheimer's/dementia can vary with each person; and even with the same person; symptoms can vary during each phase of the disease.

According to the National Institute of Health (www.nih.gov), as of 2015, Alzheimer's can only be definitively be diagnosed posthumously. A definitive diagnosis of Alzheimer's disease can be made only "through autopsy after death, by linking clinical measures with an examination of brain tissue."

However, the National Institute of Health (NIH) notes that doctors "have several methods and tools to help them determine fairly accurately whether a person who is having memory problems has 'possible Alzheimer's disease' (symptoms may be due to another cause), 'probable Alzheimer's disease' (no other cause for the symptoms can be found), or some other condition."

NIH reports that "to preliminarily diagnose Alzheimer's while the person is still living, doctors may over time:

✓ Ask questions about overall health, past medical problems, ability to carry out daily activities, and changes in behavior and personality.
✓ Conduct tests of memory, problem-solving, attention, counting, and language.
✓ Carry out standard medical tests, such as blood and urine tests, to identify other possible causes of the problem.
✓ Perform brain scans, such as computed tomography (CT/PET Scan) or magnetic resonance imaging (MRI), to distinguish Alzheimer's from other possible causes for symptoms."

On the following page, you'll find the *"Person-Centered Alzheimer's and Dementia Symptoms Tracker"* which will help you articulate the types and frequency of symptoms you are observing in your loved one and the changes you are see over time.

We recommend that you:

☐ Make 12 copies of the *Person-Centered Alzheimer's and Dementia Symptoms Tracker* from your book or for an 8.5 x 11-inch version, download this FREE tool when you visit our website: www.whencaringtakescourage.com

☐ Complete the worksheet now based upon your loved one's current symptoms.

☐ Going forward, complete a new worksheet every 30 days or when you notice significant changes so that this information can be shared with your physician, and other care providers. Recording the changes over time will help all of you to identify better and track the progression of the disease in your loved one.

Of all of the symptoms of dementia (including Alzheimer's), perhaps the most difficult for us to experience with our loved one is their gradually worsening severe memory loss.

Person-Centered Alzheimer's and Dementia Symptoms Tracker

Each person's experience with Alzheimer's or Dementia is unique to them. Symptoms may change frequently and progress differently with each person and can be affected by many factors. This tool was designed to help the family caregiver track the type and frequency of the symptoms your loved one is exhibiting to support better communication and planning with your medical team and other healthcare providers as you collaborate.

Patient Name: _____   Date of Birth: _____/_____/_____

Orientation	Daily	Weekly	Monthly	Never
Forgets name of close family and friends				
Forgets address or hometown				
Forgets date/time of year/time of day				
Asks repetitive questions				

Communication	Daily	Weekly	Monthly	Never
Has trouble using words to express needs				
Becomes frustrated when speaking				
Repeats key words/phrases/gestures				
Talks to/looks at people that aren't there				
Has difficulty with written or verbal comprehension				

Bathing and Grooming	Daily	Weekly	Monthly	Never
Refuses to change clothes				
Resists bathing (showering)				
Refuses to shave/brush teeth or hair				
Exhibits fear/anxiety regarding water or undressing				
Becomes combative during bathing or grooming				

Nutrition and Hydration	Daily	Weekly	Monthly	Never
Eats less than 1500 calories per day				
Eats more than 2500 calories per day				
Eats only a few types of food				
Eats 50% or less of meals				
Takes in less than 8 glasses of water/liquid per day				
Rapid weight loss (5 or more #'s/month)				
Rapid weight gain (5 or more #'s/month)				

Behavior	Daily	Weekly	Monthly	Never
Refuses or resists medications				
Accuses others of theft or malice				
Yells, curses or engages in name calling and/or verbally abusive				
Strikes out/throws things/hits people or things/breaks things in anger				
Fearful of new people or situations				
Disrobes inappropriately				
Exhibits sexual aggressiveness				

Judgment	Daily	Weekly	Monthly	Never
Mismanages money or bills				
Dresses inappropriately for weather or outings				
Unable to recognize potential danger				
Inability to comprehend consequences				

Engagement	Daily	Weekly	Monthly	Never
Appears anxious or fearful				
Appears sad or withdrawn				
Has difficulty making eye contact or conversation				
Demonstrates an overall lack of interest in daily life and activities				
Has difficultly self-initiating hobbies or pleasant pastimes				

Toileting	Daily	Weekly	Monthly	Never
Accidents/incontinent of urine				
Accidents/incontinent of bowel				
Attempts to "go" in places other than the toilet				
Is unaware of need to use bathroom				
In unaware when wet, soiled or has incontinent related odor				

Physical	Daily	Weekly	Monthly	Never
Has difficulty walking				
Walks with a "shuffling" gait				
Has difficulty transitioning from sitting to standing/standing to sitting				
Appears to have pain				
Changes in facial expression/drooping				
Changes in sleeping habits				
Falls (with or without injury)				
Increase in bruising/unexplained injuries				

Wandering and Safety	Daily	Weekly	Monthly	Never
Is unsafe around the stove or hot surfaces				
Is unsafe around water or faucets				
Attempts to eat things that are not food				
Has gotten lost away from home/loses caregiver on outings				
Attempts to leave home				
Is currently or still asks to drive a car				

Completed by: _____   Date Completed: _____/_____/_____

Caregivers Relationship to Patient: _____   Contact Phone: _____

Next Steps:
- ☐ Tear this page from your book or visit our website www.whencaringtakescourage.com to make copies of this form.
- ☐ Take this form to your physician/medical appointments to help guide discussions about possible treatment options and interventions.
- ☐ Update this form every 30 days or upon significant change in condition. Keep copies in dated order for your own records.

© 2014 Mara Botonis, excerpt from the book "When Caring Takes Courage". Available worldwide@: www.amazon.com

It can feel that when our loved one's short and long term memories continue to erode, so too does our opportunity to connect with them in a meaningful way. That doesn't have to be the case.

The way dementia (including Alzheimer's) impacts memory is something that researchers are still studying. What we do know, is that the more we know about our loved one's life story, the more opportunities we have to engage them in activities built around what they still can remember or appreciate at each stage in the disease process.

In Chapter 2, you'll have a chance to create a Biography to capture important parts of your loved one's life story, but first let's take a look at why this information is important as it relates to their memory loss.

Throughout our lifetime, we embark on stages of development that have their own purpose in propelling us on our life's journey. Consider the following "Memories Made over a Lifetime" chart and consider the way the important people, places, pursuits and passions change over the span of a persons' life based on what developmental stage they are in.

Important people in your life change over time. As a child, your world revolves around your parents, siblings and school friends, maybe even the people that you see in your neighborhood. As you get older, your sphere of experience grows and gradually more people enter into your immediate world. Soon your peer group and then the opposite sex become an important addition. Teachers, professors, supervisors, bosses and co-workers and leaders enter your life and occupy a position of influence. Your spouse, children and then grandchildren change your idea of immediate family as the people you live with and see everyday changes. From the Mom, who tended your skinned knee and the little brother who share your bedroom to the grandchildren that run to your open arms the important people in your life always have a special place in your heart, but time and place affect your relationships and can make some feel closer than others at times.

The same thing can happen with your sense of home. From the places you grew up, to your dormitory or barracks, your first home to your retirement home and all the places you moved in/out of and lived in between. Your idea of home, your sense of belonging and security can change as often as your address does over your lifespan.

Below you'll find *"Memories Made over a Lifetime: Typical Developmental Stages in Normal Aging"* chart with a look at how some typical developmental stages in normal aging. Take a moment and complete some of the blank squares on this chart based upon your own life:

Memories Made Over a Lifetime in Normal Aging							
	Early Childhood	In Your Teens	In Your 20's	In Your 30's	In Your 40's	In Your 50's	In Your 60's	In Your 70 +
Important People	Usually Parents, Siblings	Peers Family, teachers	Significant Other, Family, peers	Spouse, Children, Boss, Peers	Spouse, Children, Boss, Peers	Spouse, Children, Boss, Grandkids	Spouse, Children, Grandchildren Peers	Spouse, Children, Grandchildren Peers
Sense of Home	Usually Parents Home(s)	Usually Parents Home(s)	Dorm, Military Base, First Apartment	Home That is Your Choice for 1st Time	Where You Raise Your Kids, Work, Make a Life	Where Spouse Is/ Familiar Place	Where Spouse Is/ Familiar Place	Where Spouse Is/ Familiar Place
Sense of Purpose or What Drive You Each Day	Play, Learn, Experience	Explore Independence Boundaries	Establish Identity and Start Life Plan	Create Career/ Family	Contribute, Define Sense of Self	Future Focused Retirement Dreams	Reflection Lead Career Coming to Close	Legacy Driven Looking back
Favorite Music, Movies And TV								
Favorite Places, Important Events								
Pleasurable Pursuits, Hobbies, Interests								

© 2014 Mara Botonis

As we learned earlier in this chapter, dementia (including Alzheimer's) causes severe memory loss, usually most gravely impacting the short term or more recent memories. What that means is that persons with dementia have a hard time remembering things that have happened recently but may have a lot of clarity around long term memories. Life events that happen in their current and most recent decades may appear "fuzzy" while memories from their younger days seem to be more accessible.

A good example of this is when a man with dementia in his 70's tells his wife he wants to "go home" as he sits in the living room of the house he built with his own two hands and that they've lived in for 20+ years. The reason this happens is that his recent memory of home has been erased by dementia. The home he remembers, the home he longs for and wants to return to and feels safe in is the memory of a home he occupied in his past, maybe 40, 50, or 60 years ago.

Likewise, he may not currently recognize the middle-aged woman standing next to him as his daughter because, in his mind, the memories still accessible to him of his daughter are from when she was much younger, when she was a little girl.

Another common example is that our loved ones may remember the words to a song they loved in their teen years but have difficulty remembering what they ate for dinner last night.

These short term memory gaps can pose a real challenge for care partners.

There are many stories of women with dementia feeling a heart-stopping, panic-inducing visceral reaction where their blood runs cold, and the hair on the back of their neck stands up because they happen upon a strange man in their bedroom. The woman is terrified that she is experiencing a home invasion when in reality, the man is her husband. To her, this old man looks completely unfamiliar, as her husband is a handsome young man in his 30's and looks nothing like this elderly stranger who is immediately perceived as a threat.

An illustrated example of the way short term memories can be erased or "fuzzy" when dementia is present may help explain this idea. Consider the *"**Memories Made over a**

Lifetime chart again, only in this version we've added shading to represent how can dementia erode the most recently made or short-term memories. The memories that are the most difficult to retain are the newest ones-they are the "fuzziest", but with short term memory loss, the further back in someone's lifetime memories were made (these are called long-term memories), the more likely they are to be accessible as we age.

		Memories Made over a Lifetime Typical Developmental Stages Short Term Memory Loss/Dementia						
	Early Childhood	In Your Teens	In Your 20's	In Your 30's	In Your 40's	In Your 50's	In Your 60's	In Your 70 +
Important People	Usually Parents, Siblings	Peers Family, teachers	Significant Other, Family, peers	Spouse, Children, Boss, Peers	Spouse, Children, Boss, Peers	Spouse, Children, Boss, Grandkids	Spouse, Children, Grandchildren Peers	Spouse, Children, Grandchildren Peers
Sense of Home	Usually Parents Home(s)	Usually Parents Home(s)	Dorm, Military Base, First Apartment	Home That is Your Choice for 1st Time	Where You Raise Your Kids, Work, Make a Life	Where Spouse Is/ Familiar Place	Where Spouse Is/ Familiar Place	Where Spouse Is/ Familiar Place
Sense of Purpose or What Drive You Each Day	Play, Learn, Experience	Explore Independence Boundaries	Establish Identity and Start Life Plan	Create Career/ Family	Contribute, Define Sense of Self	Future Focused Retirement Dreams	Reflection Lead Career Coming to Close	Legacy Driven Looking back
Favorite Music, Movies And TV								
Favorite Places, Important Events								
Pleasurable Pursuits, Hobbies, Interests								

One of the great challenges of Alzheimer's disease is that not only are persons impacted by it subjected to the severe memory loss that impairs short-term or recent memories (like with dementia), but the plaques and tangles also create holes in the brain that gradually make more and more long-term memories inaccessible.

The shrinking of the brain and the holes in it created by plaques and tangles for persons with Alzheimer's patients makes it difficult for some long term memories to be retrieved. Depending on where each person's plaques and tangles are located within their brain, how advanced their Alzheimer's disease is, and how fast it's progressing (which are different for every person) there is no way to predict which long-term memories will "stick" and which ones will be lost, and when.

Think of the "Memories Made over a Lifetime: Short Term Memory Loss/Dementia" chart again, only this time in addition to the "fuzzy" short term memories of dementia, there are now also random holes or gaps in longer-term memories caused by the plaques and tangles of Alzheimer's disease.

Persons in the early stages of Alzheimer's disease typically have more consistent access to the parts of their memory that hold long-term memories. The people, places and times in their life that are familiar are often not in the present but found in their remote past, from a time when they were young adults or children.

This chart is just an example, for illustration. The holes or gaps in your loved one's memory will be different than what is shown on the chart as the disease impacts each person a little differently.

Next we'll learn more about how you can determine which parts of your loved one's life story is most accessible and how to incorporate those meaningful people, places and times in your loved one's past into their present day using the "failure-free" philosophy of Biography Based Care®.

Memories Made over a Lifetime
Typical Developmental Stages
Impacted by Alzheimer's

	Early Childhood	In Your Teens	In Your 20's	In Your 30's	In Your 40's	In Your 50's	In Your 60's	In Your 70 +
Important People	Usually Parents, Siblings	Peers Family, teachers	Significant Other, Family, peers	Spouse, Children, Boss, Peers	Spouse, Children, Boss, Peers	Spouse, Children, Boss, Grandkids	Spouse, Children, Grandchildren Peers	Spouse, Children, Grandchildren Peers
Sense of Home	Usually Parents Home(s)	Usually Parents Home(s)	Dorm, Military Base, First Apartment	Home That is Your Choice for 1st Time	Where You Raise Your Kids, Work, Make a Life	Where Spouse Is/ Familiar Place	Where Spouse Is/ Familiar Place	Where Spouse Is/ Familiar Place
Sense of Purpose or What Drive You Each Day	Play, Learn, Experience	Explore Independence Boundaries	Establish Identity and Start Life Plan	Create Career/ Family	Contribute, Define Sense of Self	Future Focused Retirement Dreams	Reflection Lead Career Coming to Close	Legacy Driven Looking back
Favorite Music, Movies And TV								
Favorite Places, Important Events								
Pleasurable Pursuits, Hobbies, Interests								

© 2014 Mara Botonis

CHAPTER 2

The Failure Free Philosophy of Biography Based Care®

Honey,

I need your help. Please help me have the best possible day, I may not know how anymore.

I'd really enjoy my favorite breakfast: coffee with two creamers and one sugar, toast with cinnamon and sugar sprinkled on it and a sliced banana on top of my bowl of cereal. It's nice to have the kind of breakfast I always used to start my day with when I could still make it myself. Starting with something familiar makes me feel more relaxed about embarking on the rest of our day. I used to make you breakfast sometimes. Do you remember that?

Can you help me wash my face using my favorite soap and then put lotion on my hands for me? Also, I always preferred to brush my teeth after my morning coffee, ok? Can I wear my super-soft blue sweater? It may look worn or out of fashion, but it keeps me warm, and it's easy for me to get on and off. I've had it for so long; it feels like an old friend. There are fewer and fewer things I recognize now, thank you for keeping the items I still know and remember nearby.

I know you're in a rush because you know where we need to go and what time we need to be there, but I can't remember, so please don't yell at me, ok? When your tone of voice is harsh, and your body language rushed, I retreat further into myself.

I sure like to listen to popular musical hits from my younger days and happiest times. Familiar voices and lyrics sure are nice when a large part of my day I can't understand what's being said around me. I always appreciate the chance to go outside and some gentle exercise, fresh air and feel the sun on my face. Can I walk in the yard with you, check the mail and maybe smell the fresh cut grass or flower garden? I used to be able to go wherever I wanted to whenever I wanted to.

Let me help you with something I still know how to do so I can feel useful. I used to be good at so many things. I spend big parts of my day feeling useless, forgotten, like I'm a burden that does everything wrong. I used to know how to dry tears, fix cuts and scrapes, mend broken hearts, repair damaged toys and give advice on almost everything. It may not always have been what you wanted to hear, but I always wanted the very best for you. If you want to pay me a compliment or tell me something nice, it'd sure make me feel good.

I like looking at and talking about old pictures from my childhood. I miss my parents, siblings and school days. Back when my kids were young or when we traveled together brings back some of my happiest years.

Help me fight to keep these wonderful memories and stories "fresh" in my mind by reminiscing with me often. So many life experiences are getting erased now.

I remember when dinner took a large part of the day to cook and made the house smell so good. I know the kids in our house always had to eat whatever they were served-but please skip the cooked spinach on my plate! Yuck! After we eat, I'd really like to watch some of my favorite movies, or the TV shows that I used to love; can you put one of them on for me?

Try not to wait for me to ask for help. I may not realize that I need it and it makes me feel embarrassed and bothersome to ask you. You know me so well, feel free just to do what needs to be done, I trust you to take care of me.

If I could still tell you "thank you" as often as you deserve it, to do so properly would take me thousands of hours, a millennium of minutes and dozens of days. You do so much for me. I try to tell you with the look in my eyes, my words, and my hugs, but I can't always get this brain to function like I want it to anymore.

Know this, and know it without a doubt. I love you very much. I love you as much now as I ever did. Probably 10,000 times more.

Even if those words can never be spoken on my part again, know this with certainty, I still feel the way I always have about you. My ability to tell you or show you may have been taken from me by this disease, but I still feel the way I always have about you. Nothing can rob me of that.

I'm still here. I'm right here with you.

I would give anything and everything for you to escape the hurt this is causing you too. I know it's really hard on you, and I'm sorry.

Thank you for not giving up on us.

-Me

PS. Did I mention I'd really enjoy coffee with two creamers and one sugar, toast with cinnamon and sugar sprinkled on it and a sliced banana on top of my bowl of cereal for breakfast?

Biography Based Care® is a failure free philosophy of Alzheimer's and Dementia care that is rooted in the idea that care is much more successfully provided when allowances are made that enable caregivers to tailor support to the person they are caring for based on the life experiences, favorites, and familiars of their loved one. Each person with the disease is unique. The way the disease progresses, the nature of their symptoms, the areas of strength and deficit, are all completely different at each stage of the disease and for each person. There are many resources out there that identify the stages of Alzheimer's. Many of them note that your loved one can go from one stage of the disease to another and back. Frequent changes in your loved one's behavior and abilities can occur daily and that there are many factors that can make symptoms alternately worse and sometimes better.

For years, some of the better care communities, professional practitioners, and effective family caregivers have been using parts of a person's life history to make care tasks easier for you and a lot less stressful for your loved one. At every stage in the disease process, knowing and incorporating as much of their life story as possible, is the foundation for successfully creating the best possible day for your loved one.

Using the Biography Based Care® method you'll read about here, can increase cooperation on the part of your loved one as you provide answers to the questions they may be struggling with such as: "Why would I want to do this "thing" that you're asking of me?" or "What's in it for me?" or "How is this anything like how I used to spend my day?"

The Biography Based Care® approach offers practical strategies to help you:

1. Capitalize on your loved one's current abilities and preferences.
2. Give context to daily tasks that relate back to the people, places and times in your loved one's life that are most familiar right now.
3. Provide care in a way that can decrease agitation and promote a sense of well-being and fulfillment for both of you.

For example, a common challenge many caregivers share is getting their loved one bathed. Persons with Alzheimer's/dementia may be uncomfortable with bathing for a variety of reasons including feeling vulnerable or embarrassed while undressed, confusion about why they needed to get undressed in the first place, fear of falling or even something as simple as not wanting to feel too cold or hot while wet.

Using the Biography Based Care® approach is about pre-planning, making care tasks and activities more pleasant by incorporating long-held routines identified on the personalized Biography tool provided later in this chapter. Even little things that you may not think are important can come to your aid in accomplishing care tasks just when you need it most. Details like, did your loved one normally bathe in the morning, before bedtime or both? Did they shower or take a bath? Did they do this weekly or daily? How often did your loved one wash their hair or shave? What shampoo, soap, after shave or lotions did they like to use most often? What temperature of the water is most comfortable for them? Would your loved one be more comfortable with you standing behind the shower curtain while it is drawn for privacy or do they need your help with washing in the shower/bath? What about skipping a shower altogether and using a wash basin with warm soapy water for a sponge bath?

The biography tool can help you capture the information that will be most useful to you in providing care and creating "failure-free" life enrichment activities. The Biography begins by asking you to write in some basic information about your loved one, and then guides you through different parts of your loved one's life in chronological order.

The Biography can help you identify the people, places and times in your loved one's life that are most prevalent in their stories right now. These stories are precious life experiences from your loved one's past that can be incorporated into your current caregiving routine. Using this approach can help your loved one feel more comfortable with aspects of their daily care that they may find confusing, potentially frightening or just flat out refuse to participate in.

Using pieces of the biography tool may look and sound like this: "Mom, it's time for us to wash up before church". Use of the word "wash" for shower or bath can be less frightening, and if Mom's routine in her younger days were to wash up once a week and put on clean clothes for church, this reference could evoke positive versus negative feelings around the idea of bathing. There is no need to use words like shower or tub since those may cause undue fear. Going to church after bathing is not the point, this need may be met by listening to favorite church music, reading a favored Bible passage or going out to church if your loved one is willing and able. In some cases, your loved one may not even remember the original reason for bathing after you are done washing up and that's okay. What is important is that the care task was accomplished safely with the least amount of stress created for your loved one.

How you get through these care goals, the reason "why" that you give, or the way you accomplish these can change each time you accomplish them, and that's okay, too.

Here are some quick tips to keep in mind when providing your loved one with Biography Based Care®:

☐ When starting to work on completing the Biography form in this chapter, focus on what you can answer, put as much down on paper as possible. This information may be helpful not only to you but also to other members of your care team. It's better to get started on this project sooner rather than later, as it might become more difficult to gather this information as your loved one's disease progresses, making the details that bring to life even the most important of family events more difficult to recollect.

☐ The Biography will evolve over time and really never gets finished; you will always be adding or changing it as you remember things you'll want to add as your loved one's preferences change. The biography form included for you on the following pages is designed to help get you started. Complete as much of it as you can, capture what you know and ask other family members for help. It's okay if you can't answer every question and it's okay to give yourself some time to complete. Some families like to do a little each day, others divide up different parts, and some families make it an activity by engaging their loved one in reminiscing. Do your best to make it as complete as possible while forgiving yourself for any gaps. Use what you know, combined with the tips in this book to support your caregiving efforts in the best possible way.

☐ A wonderful window into the world your loved one may sometimes retreat to comes from their words and actions if you know how to interpret them. It may sometimes seem that they are not looking at you or even seeing you, not listening to you or being "present" with you in the realm of reality. Listen to the stories they tell again and again for clues as to the people, places and times in their life that are still accessible experiences for them. Jot down notes of names and words they use, pictures or objects they seem to show an interest in or times when their behavior or mood changes for the better so you can seek to incorporate those elements into their day more often.

☐ Integrating familiar people. A common source of agitation or restlessness may be the result of your loved one looking for a person that is not available. For example, your loved one may ask or look for their mother, though she's been gone for years. Identifying favorite foods, holiday traditions or other memories related to your loved one's early days on the Biography will then help you create ways to incorporate the idea of her in everyday activities. For example, "It's Sunday, and that means pot roast for dinner with your Mother's homemade gravy recipe" or "Let's string popcorn for the Christmas tree like you did with your Mom", or "Smell these beautiful roses. I know your Mom had a wonderful rose garden in the front yard when you lived in the house by the creek". Integrating sights, sounds, smells, textures and tastes that evoke memories of a favorite person can be a terrific way to engage your loved one in activities that meet a variety of needs.

☐ Incorporating favorite places can seem like a challenge, especially when the place that your loved one longs for in their memory, the one that stays forever frozen in time just as they remembered it, may be long gone. The key to re-creating the place is to focus on the feelings that the place evokes. When your loved one aches for a particular place, it's often an indicator that there is an unmet underlying need. For example, they may repeat, "I want to go home" even when they are sitting in the living room of the house they've lived in for years. Use the biography to help you extract forgotten details about what they or others in their family remember about places they've lived over the years. Was there a porch swing? Did they like to eat with their family at the picnic table on a warm day? Was there a tree with a tire swing? Did it always smell like honeysuckle when the wind blew? Was their room decorated in movie posters or aircraft memorabilia? Learning more about those things that evoke a sense of home can help you re-create the feelings associated with the place. When most of us think of home, it's a place that you were always welcomed with open arms, a place where you felt a sense of safety and belonging, a place you felt loved and important. Incorporating some of these physical reminders or photos of home can help you create, and your loved one reminisce about a time before Alzheimer's/dementia when their whole world was encapsulated in a favorite neighborhood.

☐ Talking about a particular time in their life? Does your loved one often talk about their time in the military? Bring up memories of when their kids were babies? Relive past travels, jobs or events repeatedly? Taking frequent virtual "trips" to the past can be another indicator that there may be unmet needs in the present. Use the biography to learn as much as you can about what it was about the times your loved one keeps re-living that are most meaningful. Again focus on feelings, not the facts. Their need to revisit those eras may come from a desire to re-experience times that evoke positive feeling associated with a sense of accomplishment, being needed, capable and contributing. Find ways to let them take the lead, ask their advice, praise their efforts and engage them in activities and reminiscing that bring those past positive experiences right into the present. Sometimes the reflection is about wanting to define their legacy which is a developmental stage and a natural part of the aging process. Persons with Alzheimer's/dementia have the same need, especially in the early stages of the disease, to define what their life "has been about" or how they might be remembered. Sometimes retreating to the past can stem from a desire to resolve past conflict or hurt. Ask them to tell you more, and listen for clues as to what they may be missing most so you can work to provide it. Writing letters, asking them to share with you what they wished they would've said or done can help when there is a need for closure. Seek first to understand the "Why?" behind your loved one's proclivity for the past and then you can identify ways to push it forward into the present.

☐ Preferences are important. Think about having a hamburger for example. I can't remember ever seeing any two people eat a burger the same way. No mustard, no pickles, no raw onions. Add mayonnaise, ketchup, tomatoes, lettuce, cheese, crisp bacon and sautéed mushrooms. Chances are I lost a few of you somewhere along the way with that hamburger order. If I served a hamburger to everyone the way I liked it, not everyone would eat it, and some wouldn't even taste it. Imagine being at a barbecue where all you were served at every meal were things you didn't like, prepared in a manner that you didn't think tasted good. To top it off, someone else may have even dressed you in an outfit you found tight, too hot and made from an itchy material. Now, how much fun are you having? Person's with Alzheimer's/dementia may not be as able to articulate their own needs anymore and as a result of being in situations that aren't to their liking, they may act out or fail to extract the maximum benefit. If they are dressed in uncomfortable clothing, for example, that may be one reason they keep shedding their shoes or pants. If their food is served in a way that doesn't taste good to your loved one, that could explain part of the weight loss and decrease in appetite. The Biography can help you capture all of the preferences that make your loved one unique and that you are now responsible for honoring and protecting because they can no longer do so. Doing things the way they always have, or prefer can help increase cooperation, create positive outcomes and decrease disruptive behavior so it's well worth your time (for a lot of reasons) to incorporate their preferences any way you can. It's also a great way to show them you care.

☐ Look for what works and continue to try different ideas that are not bound by "the way it's supposed to be done" necessarily but are created anew each time based on what your loved one can and wants to do at the moment. Use that to guide them in accomplishing the task or enjoying the activity at hand. Who says "playing cards" requires rules and a certain method of play. Sorting by suit, putting in numeric order and even holding the cards while snacking on veggies and homemade dip can be enough to re-create the positive parts of card play from the past. Focus on what your loved one can do and build the adapted version of reminiscing, a favorite hobby, or activity of daily living around those abilities, minimizing the deficits.

☐ Success lies in looking for and recognizing the positives. This approach is all about translating old favorites, familiar pastimes, long-held routines and past preferences into activities that engage your loved one and create the best possible day. The more you know about them, the more you'll have to work with when it comes to brainstorming new ways to bring the "old days" forward.

So, grab a cup of coffee, tea or a favorite beverage, sit in a comfortable chair, and remove the Biography pages from the book. Yes, I said rip pages out of the book. Yes, it's okay. *When Caring Takes Courage* is YOUR book, and there are lots of places I'm going to encourage you to take pages out and use them, write in the spaces provided, take your completed pages with you to physician appointments, or dog-ear pages that are of interest to you. *When Caring Takes Courage* is a book that is meant to be USED, not just READ. If it just sits on your shelf and collects dust, I've done you a grave disservice, so please feel free to consider it a workbook of sorts.

We also have a copy of the Biography form you can print and save on our website: www.whencaringtakescourage.com.

Now back to the Biography, remove the Biography pages from your book and keep them handy. Whenever you can sneak in a few minutes here or there, start jotting down what you do know and ask others for their memories if your loved one is unable to answer your questions. The more information you can gather and share on this biography, the more approaches and ideas you'll have to draw upon when you most need them to support your loved one.

Biography ❦ Based Care®

Biography Template

Loved one's Full Name		Likes to be Called		Date of Birth	
Primary Caregiver Name		Relationship to Person with Dementia		Caregiver phone number	

Wears glasses/reading glasses	Yes	No	Wears hearing aid(s)		Yes	No
Wears upper/lower dentures	Yes	No	Wears incontinence product daytime		Yes	No
Uses walker/cane	Yes	No	Wears incontinence product nighttime		Yes	No
Uses wheelchair	Yes	No	Diabetic		Yes	No

Early Childhood/Young Adulthood (Birth to 17 years old)　　　Years: 19____ to 19____

Parents' names	Mom: Dad:
Grandparents names	Grandmothers: Grandfathers:
Siblings' names. and birth order (from oldest to youngest including your loved one)	Note: sister or brother:
Pet names and type of animal(s)	
Name of elementary and high schools attended, city and state of each. Any specific school age memories	
Home-city, state and memories of houses, yard, neighborhood	
Favorite hobbies, music/songs, sports & leisure activities at this age	
Favorite holiday traditions at this age	
Trips or vacations during this era	
Faith based activities (name of church, favorite verses or hymns etc.)	
Family car, first car	
Notable personal history, or significant events, best friend(s) at this age	

© 2014 Mara Botonis, excerpt from the book, "When Caring Takes Courage" available worldwide on amazon.com

Early Adulthood *(18 to 50 years old)*   Years: 19_____ to 19_____

Spouse or significant other names	Full name: Likes to be called:
Date(s) married and length of marriage	
Courtship: when where, typical dates, how they met and anything about this era that evokes pleasant feelings	
Children's names and birth order from oldest to youngest and place of residence currently Note: son or daughter	
Routines at this age: dressing, grooming, sleeping and eating habits	
Work or career during this era — be specific about company, role, duties	
Military Service during this era. Specific about branch of service, length of service, war(s) served in (if any), military job, where stationed, if retired (when), etc.	
Name of college attended (if any), city and state of each, area of study, degree(s) received, specific college era memories	
Home-city, state and memories of houses, yard, neighborhood	
Favorite hobbies, music/songs, sports/leisure activities at this age	
Favorite holiday traditions from this era	
Trips or vacations during this time frame	
Faith based activities (name of church, personal involvement role, such as usher, choir), favorite verses/hymns)	
Notable personal history, or significant events at this age	

Late Adulthood *(50 to present years old)*   Years: 19_____ to: Present

Names of grandchildren from oldest to youngest	
Routines during this time; dressing, grooming, sleeping and eating habits	
Work or career during this era — be specific about company, role, duties, general dates of employment. For retirement years, describe a typical day	
Home-city, state and memories of houses, yard, neighborhood	
Favorite hobbies, music/songs, sports or leisure activities during this time frame	
Favorite holiday traditions at this age	
Favorite trips or vacations during this era	
Faith based activities (name of church, personal involvement role, favorite verses or hymns etc.)	
Notable personal history, or significant events at this age	

Favorites and Familiars   (past and present)

Shampoo/Soap Aftershave Lotion Toothpaste	
Morning routine – what time usually Rises? Shower? Shave? Exercise? Breakfast?	
Bathing preference (bath or shower, am or pm, how frequently)	
Hair Style (how do they like to wear it, have it styled, how often cut)	
Facial care Make up (what and how) or shaving (electric or razor, how and when)	
Evening routine – Watch TV? Read? Listen to Music? Toileting (brush teeth, wash face etc.)? When is bedtime?	
Sleeping habits/patterns – typical length of nighttime sleep? Naps during day? Night light? Able to go to toilet alone?	
Breakfast food and drink – what is a typical breakfast meal for your loved one and what time do they usually eat it?	
Lunch food and drink – what types of items (sandwiches, soups, fruit?) does your loved one usually have for lunch and about what time?	
Dinner food and drink – what is a normal dinner meal for your loved one? What time is it usually served?	

© 2014 Mara Botonis, excerpt from the book, "When Caring Takes Courage" available worldwide on amazon.com

Desserts – what are examples of your loved one's favorites (fruit, ice cream, cookies, pies, cakes – what kind)?	
Snacks – what are some favorite snack foods (popcorn, fruit or vegetables, cookies, cheese and crackers) and beverages (coffee, tea, lemonade, fruit juice, milk)?	
What is your loved one used to wearing every day – what is easiest for this person to get in and out of?	
Preferred sleeping attire – what does your loved one normally wear to bed (pajamas or nightgown, sweatpants, shorts)?	
Favorite types of shows, specific movies/ TV shows or favorite stars – what kinds of programs does your loved one enjoy?	
Favorite place(s) – what are some of the places your loved one enjoyed or enjoys visiting the most?	
The people, places and times in their life that are most often mentioned (currently)	
The times of day or specific activities that are most engaging (currently) for your loved one are;	
The most effective ways to comfort your loved one when they are sad, angry or upset:	

© 2014 Mara Botonis, excerpt from the book, "When Caring Takes Courage" available worldwide on amazon.com

Additional Biographical Notes:

Completed by: _____   Contact Phone #: _____

Relationship to patient: _____   Date: _____

Completed by: _____   Contact Phone #: _____

Relationship to patient: _____   Date: _____

CHAPTER 3

Communicating with Care

People with Alzheimer's and Dementia may have trouble both comprehending and using language. The decreased ability to communicate may cause frustration and lead to embarrassment, anxiety and even aggressiveness. Changes in your loved one's ability to communicate can vary and are based on where he or she is in the disease process. At different stages of dementia, you may notice these changes in your loved one's ability to communicate:

- ✓ Difficulty finding the right words to accurately convey their message.
- ✓ Using familiar words repeatedly in place of the "right" word(s).
- ✓ Describing familiar objects to you rather than calling them by name.
- ✓ Losing their train of thought mid-sentence/mid-story.
- ✓ Difficulty organizing words logically, the "correct" words are written or spoken out of order.
- ✓ Speaking less often out of embarrassment, fear or uncertainty.
- ✓ Relying on physical gestures rather than speaking.

Communication is critical in any relationship, but especially so when it comes to communicating with a person who has signs and symptoms of Alzheimer's/Dementia. Communication is an important tether that can connect your loved one to you, to others and the world around them.

As changes occur over time, your loved one's ability to communicate will as well. When we think of how we communicate with others, we might first reflect on what we say or read. Often I hear from families that their loved one is no longer able to communicate, but what they might really mean, is that their loved one is not as able to talk with them as they used to. The good news, based upon what we now know, is that despite eroding verbal communication skills over the course of progressive types of dementia, we still have a lot of ways to connect with our loved ones.

What's surprising is that according to www.nonverbalgroup.com, "is that 93% of all daily communication is nonverbal. Dr. Albert Mehrabian, the author of Silent Messages, conducted several studies on nonverbal communication. He found that only 7% of ANY message is conveyed through words, 38% through certain vocal elements, and 55% through nonverbal elements (facial expressions, gestures, posture, etc.). Subtracting the 7% for actual vocal content leaves one with the 93% statistic. The studies concluded that 93% of ALL communication is actually non-verbal."

The tips below may help you better communication with your loved one.

- ☐ Do strive to be patient. Let your loved one take their time trying to find the right words. Don't rush to fill in the rest of the sentence or assume you know the point they are trying to make before they finish. You can decrease frustration for both of you by giving each other ample time to gather your thoughts and ideas before trying to express them.

- ☐ Do strive to be supportive and encouraging. Let your loved one know, "it's okay" and tell them to "take your time". Demonstrate your sincere interest in what they are trying to communicate by maintaining eye contact, avoiding distractions, and using body language, including reassuring touch.

- ☐ Don't make assumptions about your loved one's ability to communicate because of an Alzheimer's diagnosis or symptoms of dementia. The disease affects each person differently.

- ☐ Don't leave your loved one out of conversations by talking to others as if they weren't there. Coach others in your life to keep trying to engage your loved one in reaching out in a variety of ways when trying to communicate.

☐ Do ask others to speak directly to your loved one versus asking you how they are doing. When your loved one is part of a conversation they may have difficulty participating in, offer a smile or reassuring pat on the hand and make eye contact. These are all ways to let your loved one know that they are an important part of the conversation even though they may have difficulty contributing.

☐ Do give your loved one time to respond. Try to avoid interrupting or finishing their sentences. Your loved one might just need a little more time to "find" their words. Your patience will pay off as you help your loved one feel that they have something to say and that you really want to hear them. Giving them the time they need to gather their thoughts and express their ideas can also decrease frustration on their part due to their perception that they need to "hurry" and speak before someone cuts them off or decides for them what they were trying to say.

☐ Do listen for feelings, not facts. Often person's with Alzheimer's/dementia may substitute words and phrases or repeat certain words again and again. Instead of listening to the actual word choices, search to understand the intention. Try not to correct or criticize your loved one.

☐ Do use body language. Pointing, gesturing, and touch can help both you and your loved one get your point across effectively by "showing" each other what you mean when it's difficult to "say" it.

☐ Do identify your loved one's preferred sense(s). We all process information differently and the same is true for a person with Alzheimer's/dementia. Noticing if your loved one does better with things they see, hear, taste, smell or touch can help you communicate with them in the way that they can be most successful by sharing information using their preferred sense(s).

☐ Do try to keep it simple. Use short sentences, with clear and simple subjects. Don't ask "How?" "When?" or "Why?" which are more conceptual or intangible questions that your loved one may have difficulty processing. Talk slowly, and clearly. Go one step at a time when giving directions. Repeat as needed.

☐ Do make decision making easy. Offering just a choice of two things makes conveying their choices less overwhelming. Instead of asking open-ended questions, try giving a choice of just two options to empower your loved one to participate in decision-making in a way that is more manageable for them.

☐ Do avoid arguing. When you feel or see either of you getting frustrated, take a deep breath and pause. Agitation can escalate quickly, and your tone of voice, the pace of the conversation and word choices may unintentionally cause negative consequences for both of you.

☐ Your loved one takes cues from your demeanor. Even when things are frustrating for you both, try to convey a sense of calm to avoid escalating things any further.

☐ Do keep your focus on the outcome. Keep in mind the desired outcome and how you can best accomplish it. Keeping the goal in mind can help you avoid getting caught up in details that don't matter in the grand scheme of things.

☐ Do offer a guess at times. Due to the changes in their brain, your loved one's ability to use and comprehend language may be impacted. They may use the wrong word at the wrong time or substitute a still familiar word for many that they cannot remember. When you feel like it may be helpful, you may support them in communication by offering interpretations of what they may be trying to say. We recommend that this done respectfully and after they feel that they've been given enough time to express themselves without interruption.

☐ Do encourage non-verbal communication. Use your tone of voice, facial expressions, body language and gentle touch to guide or reassure your loved one.

☐ Do try to limit distractions. Find a place that's quiet. If television, radio, or background noise is present, it can be more difficult for your loved one to concentrate. The surroundings should support your loved one's ability to focus on their thoughts. Create a quiet, peaceful place with limited auditory distractions or busy visual stimulation.

☐ Consider using pictures to help your loved one make their point. Simple line drawings or clip art from the internet with pictures of water, a meal, a toilet or other simple images may help your loved one articulate their needs. If you don't understand what your loved one is trying to tell you, ask them to point or "show you" what they are trying to say.

☐ Do be open to recognizing and encouraging different types of communication. Often as the disease progresses, you may find that your loved one seems to respond better using one of their five senses or another (or a combination) at different stages. Try to engage their sense of sight, smell, hearing, taste, and touch to increase the chances that your message may "get through" to them. For example, your loved one may simply offer a smile or nod when they can no longer say the things they want to. A person may simply rhythmically pat their thigh when enjoying a song long after their ability to sing along is gone.

☐ Do endeavor to be forgiving. Things aren't always going to go as you'd have liked and there will be times that hurtful things may be said. Try not to take things personally and agree to forgive yourself and your loved one when things don't go as planned. Remember, it's okay to "start over" and come back to the conversation with a fresh perspective, attitude and approach.

☐ It's OK if you don't know what to do or say in every situation. Sometimes, while caring for a person with Alzheimer's/dementia, you may hear or your see things that are difficult to make sense of, keep in mind that your love, your very presence and an environment free from the fear of failure are what's most important to your loved one. When in doubt, choose a reassuring word or phrase versus judging or correcting.

CHAPTER 4
Bathing without Battling

For persons with Alzheimer's /dementia bathing can be a frightening and stressful time. Bathing is also commonly cited as the hardest care task that caregivers (both professional and family members) need to accomplish.

The decreased ability to communicate, comprehend what is happening and the "why" of having to get undressed, feel cold, embarrassed or vulnerable during the phases of bathing. Feeling frustrated by a perceived lack of privacy or forced dependence on another person for such an intimate task can be very difficult for your loved one. The disease process itself can also work against you as it may also increase their sensitivity to the amount of warmth in the water, the temperature of the room while dressing/undressing, the way the water feels on their body and the pressure it creates when it touches fragile skin. All of these factors can lead your loved one down a path of resistance, agitation, and potential aggressiveness. Persons living with Alzheimer's/dementia may be more likely to resist bathing by yelling or engaging in verbally abusive behavior, or even striking out during the process. This behavior can occur for a variety of reasons, but the tips below can help you increase the chance of preventing these behaviors before they start.

BEFORE BATHING

□ Lower the thermostat on your hot-water heater to prevent scalding injuries, and always check the temperature of the water yourself to ensure that it's safe.

□ Make safety your number one priority. Evaluate and minimize potential risks before you begin assisting your loved one with shower/bathing. Engage your loved one's physician in conversations about how best to decrease the risk of falls and utilize any recommendations for adaptive equipment that help increase both safety and comfort, such as: a hand-held shower head, grab bars at different heights, a shower bench, bath chair or tub seat, non-slip bath mats, etc. Purchase blue and red colored circle shaped stickers from your local office supply store and affix the stickers to the tops of all of the water faucets in the house, red on the hot water faucet, blue on the cold water faucet to decrease confusion between the two.

☐ Be understanding. Bathing is often one of the activities of daily living that can cause the greatest amount of stress for persons with Alzheimer's/dementia and their caregivers. Your loved one may be fearful of falling, uneasy about getting undressed, confused by the need to bathe, or even afraid of the water and the sounds and feelings of different textures associated with bathing. Noticing which aspects of bathing are most stressful for your loved one can help you problem solve more effectively. When they exhibit fear or discomfort, take note of what is happening in that moment for them and then:

☐ Be prepared. Gather all needed supplies BEFORE you start the bathing process and place them within easy reach. Bath time preparation should include not only toiletries and items needed for bathing but also a clean set of towels and change of clothes.

☐ Plan ahead. There are many sequential steps in the bathing process that may be confusing to your loved one. The vulnerable feeling that may accompany getting undressed and dressed can also cause this process to take more time or an unpredictable amount of time from bath to bath. Try to accomplish bathing when you have twice as much time as you think you'll need to complete the task to avoid feeling rushed.

☐ Have your loved one prepare to bathe independently as much as possible (safely). Set your loved one up to do pieces of bathing independently whenever possible. Have a shower bench, hand-held shower, non-slip mats and a warm, soapy washcloth to help your loved one participate more in washing themselves while you stand by for safety. Give verbal cues, and point to areas on you that your loved one needs to wash (if needed).

☐ Ensure comfort. Be sure to run water and test it yourself before you invite them to get wet to ensure a comfortable temperature before your loved one steps in as they may not be able to tell you if it is too hot or too cold. Put towels and clothing in the dryer before you get your loved one into the shower/bath so the fabric has been gently warmed and is ready to wrap your loved one up cozily when they get dried off and dressed.

WHILE WASHING

☐ Never leave your loved one without appropriate supervision in the bathroom. In addition to the risks of scalding, flooding, slipping or falling; there are often hidden dangers such as: ingesting non-edible cleaning and grooming supplies or flooding the house because they may forget to turn the water off. It's a fine line between protecting their sense of privacy and ensuring their safety, when in doubt, safety first.

☐ Protect their dignity and privacy. Have a towel or washcloth for them to hold and keep areas you are not actively washing or rinsing covered to help them maintain both warmth and privacy.

☐ Honor preferences. Try to replicate the way your loved one would have gone about these tasks by taking into consideration when and how they did these tasks for themselves. Washing in the same order (i.e. shave before or after the shower?) your loved one always did. Use the same soaps and shampoos and notice previous bathing patterns (e.g. did they use the shower or bath in the tub? Bathe once a day or once a week? Bathe before bed or in the morning?). These thoughtful considerations can help to create a sense of the familiar for your loved one.

- Check for signs of pain or irritation weekly. Look for redness, bruising or evidence of favoring or wincing when moving certain parts of their body or being touched. Identify and communicate with your loved one's physician about any changes in skin condition or sites of potential injury or pain. If your loved one is incontinent of bowel or bladder, make sure their genital areas are cleaned and dried thoroughly to decrease the likelihood of skin breakdown. Other areas prone to skin irritation are any places where skin folds occur and under the breasts, so make sure to clean and dry those parts too. To protect fragile skin, use a gentle cleanser and avoid harsh exfoliating bath products or wash cloths.

- Be flexible. The main goal is to promote hygiene and health safely. It's okay to let your loved one go into a bath or shower fully clothed or in their bathing suit if that makes them feel more comfortable and less embarrassed. Be okay with getting wet yourself if that's what it takes! Also, be open to using waterless shampoo, washing your loved one's hair in the sink or beauty parlor, using baby wipes/sponge baths instead of shower or tub bath. You can also try different times of the day or different days of the week until you get a routine established that seems to work well.

- Offer cues in a couple of different ways. For example, when giving verbal instructions, use simple phrases like: "wash your arm with this washcloth" or "sit down here". You can also try to help your loved one with the "hand over hand" technique by placing your hand atop theirs and guiding them by moving your hands together to complete the required action. A third technique is "modeling" the desired action by showing them how to do it by performing the task yourself while they observe and then mimic what you are doing. In this example, both of you would wear your bathing suits while you wash yourself one step at a time, and then your own hair, pausing throughout to give them time to complete the process on themselves.

- Be sure to engage your loved one in decision making and ask them to make a choice between two things often to help them maintain a sense of control and independence. Asking things like, "Would you like to wash your hair or feet first?" or "Which washcloth do you like better (while letting them see and touch both examples) are great ways to let your loved one know that they are still "in charge". Ask them to smell the shampoo, hold a washcloth or the soap to give them an important task and distraction.

☐ Communicate clearly ahead of time. Let your loved one know what you'll be doing BEFORE you do it to decrease surprise and fright. "Mom, I'm going to wash your back now" or "Honey, I'm going to put shaving cream on your face" can help your loved one prepare for your touch.

☐ Offer encouragement all along the way. Reassuring words and phrases to let your loved one know that they are doing a good job, that they are almost done or that their hair smells good, their fingernails look really clean, etc. can help boost confidence and level of comfort in an otherwise potentially stressful circumstance. Look for chances to praise and recognize them for their help and cooperation.

BRINGING CLEANING TO A CLOSE

☐ Let your loved one wrap up in a bath size towel that offers maximum warmth and coverage to help then feel more comfortable while you pat them dry (versus rubbing) as they sit down to decrease the risk of falling.

☐ Make sure areas prone to skin breakdown/infection and that are likely to retain moisture such as ears, in between toes, underneath breasts and genitals are dried carefully and covered in talcum powder or cornstarch before assisting your loved one in getting dressed.

☐ Apply hypo-allergenic aromatherapy lotion to keep skin soft and create a calming post bathing experience. Scents can be general such as lavender, bergamot, lemon balm can evoke pleasant memories for your loved one specifically by using a favorite and familiar scent like that of a certain flower, plant or place (ocean, mountains, meadow, etc.) Look at a bath product specialty stores for a great variety of scents.

☐ Restore a feeling of relaxation by playing favorite soothing music, offering a warm beverage or rewarding with a favorite snack and giving your loved one some space to sit quietly or relax a moment before going on to your next activity together.

CHAPTER 5

Dressing and Grooming Made Easier

People with Alzheimer's disease often need more time to dress as sequential or multi-step tasks become more challenging. It can be hard for your loved one to choose their clothes, as they might wear the wrong clothing for the season, wear colors that don't go together or forget to put on a piece of clothing, or even put it on the wrong way (wearing a bra on top of instead of under a blouse for example). They may not remember what a toothbrush is for or why clipping their nails is important. There are many reasons why having strategies for successful grooming and dressing support are important. First, maintaining good personal hygiene, including wearing clean undergarments, can help decrease the risk of a urinary tract or other infection that might further complicate care. Secondly, when people feel good about how they look, they often feel better about themselves. For some, grooming is less about self-esteem and more about maintaining a set routine. For others, it's a task fraught with strife and undertaken only when necessary to reduce the risk of disease or infection. In any case, helping persons with Alzheimer's disease engage in grooming and dressing is an ongoing and important part of caregiving.

☐ Let your loved one do as much as possible themselves for as long as possible to foster a sense of accomplishment and involvement. Set up all supplies ahead of time (i.e. fill a small cup with mouthwash for rinsing or pre-soap a washcloth for wiping faces). For dressing, simplify a closet full of overwhelming options by offering a choice between just two already complete outfits from head to toe. Lay clothing out in the order that they will be donned, such as underwear and bra first, and then shirts and pants or, first the toothbrush with toothpaste on it and then the cup with mouthwash in it.

☐ Demonstrate the grooming task that you'd like them to perform. Brushing your own hair or teeth, washing your own face or mimicking the act of shaving can cue your loved one as to what it is they should be doing. Give step by step instructions, but one at a time. "First, let's both put the toothbrush in our mouth" and then "move the toothbrush up and down over our teeth".

☐ Use the right tools. For example, if your loved one has difficulty performing the circular motion needed to brush their teeth, try an electric toothbrush, If the sound of an electric toothbrush is intimidating for them, try using oral care swabs available for purchase at most pharmacies. Same goes for shaving, try an electric razor, or their preferred type of razor, such as disposable, quad head, etc. When shaving becomes difficult, consider having the barber help during regular visits.

☐ Take over responsibility for tasks that come with the risk of injury or infection if not done properly. Cleaning dentures, in some cases shaving, and cutting toe and fingernails are some examples of grooming tasks that may be more safely and thoroughly accomplished by you.

☐ Maintain their usual or familiar grooming routines. If your loved one has always gone to their beauty shop or a barber, continue to do so for as long as possible. If the experience becomes too distressing, it may be possible to have the barber or hairstylist come to your home.

☐ Use your loved one's favorite toiletries. Allow them to continue using their favorite soap, shampoo, toothpaste, shaving cream, cologne or makeup. These familiar smells, labels, and textures may provide a sense of comfort during what can become a stressful time of day.

☐ Allow twice as much time as you think you'll need. Rushing your loved one can cause anxiety and frustration that may result in aggressive behavior. Also, be flexible on when grooming tasks are accomplished. Trying to get your loved one bathed, dressed, groomed and fed along with morning medications in BEFORE a morning doctor's appointment may be a difficult proposition. Shaving the night before, or clipping nails in the evening may save valuable time in the morning and allow for a more relaxed and stress-free pace when it comes to the parts of grooming that are best done in the morning.

☐ Praise often and keep the environment positive and calm. While it's important to limit distractions, you may notice that your loved one has a more relaxed grooming experience with their favorite music on or with the local news on in the background. Try engaging other senses, such as smell by putting on a freshly brewed pot of coffee if these things were a normal part of their routine.

☐ Simplify choices. Pack clothes away that aren't worn as often to reduce the number of choices. Keep only a couple of outfits in the closet or dresser. Buy three or four sets of the same clothes if your loved one wants to wear the same clothing repeatedly. Try putting on one hanger whole outfits from top to bottom including socks, undergarments and shoes that can be hung in bags over the neck of the hanger. Having these "grab and go" outfits all together will make things easier for you both. Put away all inappropriate clothes and shoes when your loved one is asleep or resting to help facilitate better choices when they look in their closet.

☐ Pick comfortable and simple clothing. Cardigans, shirts or blouses that button in front are much easier to work than pullover tops. Substitute Velcro® for buttons, snaps or zippers, which may be too difficult for your loved one to handle. Make sure that clothing is not too tight and fits loosely, especially at the waist and hips. Choose fabrics that are soft and stretchable so they don't irritate the skin or feel constrictive. Make sure your loved one has comfortable, non-slip shoes with rubber soles and low heals. Buy loose-fitting, comfortable clothing, such as sports bras, cotton socks and underwear, sweatpants and shorts with elastic waistbands.

☐ Be flexible. The rule of thumb for deciding whether or not to intervene is "can potential harm come to my loved one?" If the answer is "No", then go with the flow. It's all right if they want to wear several layers of clothing, just make sure your loved one doesn't get too cold or overheated. When outdoors, make sure they are dressed appropriately for the weather.

CHAPTER 6
Toileting Tips and "Accident" Prevention

Incontinence or "accidents" are often cited as a common source of stress for the primary caregiver and embarrassment and agitation for the person with Alzheimer's/dementia.

Here are some practical solutions for this everyday challenge:

- ☐ In the early stages, make it easy for your loved one to find a bathroom. Put a picture of a toilet on the outside of the bathroom door to make it easier for them to recognize where the restroom is and the purpose of the room. At night time, make sure the pathway to the bathroom is clear and there is adequate light. Consider a night-light in the bathroom.

- ☐ Your loved one may not recognize the need to use the toilet, "suggestions" to go to the bathroom can be very helpful. Begin a toileting routine early on in the disease process. Remind and offer to escort your loved one to the bathroom when they first wake up, every two hours during the day, and especially before bedtime. Remember the mantra "more bathroom breaks equals fewer accidents."

- ☐ As dementia progresses, there usually comes a time in mid to later stages when your loved one is not aware that they need to go to the bathroom. Look for signs they may need to use the toilet. They may tug at their clothing, fidget, pace, or even start to wander.

- ☐ Accidents will occur. Try be calm and understanding as your loved one will likely be embarrassed enough already.

☐ Wear gloves to help prevent the spread of disease; washing hands before and after providing toileting assistance reduces the risk of infection.

☐ If your loved one is cognitively or physically unable use the toilet, urinal, commode, or bedpan, incontinence products will be necessary.

☐ Watch for signs of urinary tract infection or (blood in urine, cloudy urine with sediment, or dehydration (urine that is dark in color or has a strong odor, etc.) and be sure to share with your doctor if those signs are present.

☐ A person with middle-stage Alzheimer's disease (AD) cannot toilet themselves independently. Some caregivers will wake the person at night to take him to the bathroom while others prefer to use incontinence products.

☐ Alzheimer's and dementia often mean your loved one will begin to have difficulty using the bathroom and at some stage in the disease process, you'll likely need to use incontinence products. Usually, this will start to occur in the middle to late stages of the disease and can be caused by the loss of ability to recognize the urge to go, losing control of the muscles responsible for regulating bowel and bladder.

☐ There are many types and brands of incontinence products available, but there generally fall into three main types of products. There are male guards that are similar to sanitary napkins. They fit in the front of men's underwear and will catch urine. There are pull-up briefs that look a lot like regular underwear. Pull-up type briefs work best if your loved one is still able to get around the house. The last type of incontinence products are the adult diapers. Adult diapers are designed to be easier to put on or take off of your loved one when they are either bed-ridden or unable to bear weight/stand up.

☐ When the loss of bladder control begins, you will need to take extra measures to keep the genital area clean because excess moisture is present. Disposable wipes are the easiest to use and can be thrown away ensuring a clean wipe each time while not increasing your laundry pile. Take extra care to ensure your loved one has clean, dry clothes on and offer trips to the bathroom often to prevent "accidents" before they occur.

☐ When assisting your loved one with toileting or changing, be sure to look for reddened areas that may be an early indicator of potential skin breakdown, infection or discomfort. There are lots of ointments and lotions on the market that can help protect your loved one's sensitive skin as incontinence occurs. Check with your doctor or pharmacist for recommendations.

☐ To help protect your mattress, consider a waterproof mattress cover, cloth bed pads with a built-in moisture barrier that can be placed under fitted sheet and disposable bed pads that can be used on top of the sheets. The goal again is to both keep your loved one as clean and dry as possible while managing the volume of laundry that incontinence brings with it.

☐ It is rare for a person in the middle or late stages of Alzheimer's/dementia to make it through the night without wetting. You may want to cut down on fluids later in the evening. If you do, make sure they are still getting plenty of fluids during the day.

CHAPTER 7

Important Nutrition and Hydration Solutions

Changes in appetite are a common occurrence in those with Alzheimer's/dementia for a variety of reasons. For example, mealtimes can be an over-stimulating experience for person's with Alzheimer's/dementia, your loved one may not recognize that the items on their plate are edible, they may have difficulty with the senses of taste and smell that many of us rely on to make dining more enjoyable. Your loved one may have other physical factors negatively impacting their appetite also, such as lack of physical exercise, adverse reactions to medications or even potential dental problems such as poorly fitting dentures. Making a few easy adjustments may help you meet your loved one's nutritional needs more successfully and may help decrease the risk of malnutrition and/or dehydration.

- ☐ Always provide adequate supervision. Your loved one may have difficulty swallowing, may forget to chew their bites enough before attempting to swallow or forget to take in enough fluid during meals. All of these can lead to an increased risk of choking. Stay close by when your loved one is eating and be sure to familiarize yourself with the Heimlich maneuver before you may need to use it.

- ☐ Check your loved one's mouth for any areas that appear sore, look to see if there is an open wound and ask them as you gently swab their mouth if it hurts anywhere. Make note of any dental discomfort or swallowing difficult then report these to your dentist and physician.

- ☐ Contact your loved one's primary care physician and let them know about their decreased appetite. Be sure to have ready a list of all current medication and any vitamin supplements that your loved one is taking for their doctor to review.

☐ Track intake and changes in weight and/or appetite weekly if you suspect that there are significant changes in weight. Record your loved one's weight monthly and communicate any weight changes of over 5 pounds per month to the physician. Notice how much of their meals your loved one consumes on average as this can also help you and your doctor evaluate the need for nutritional supplements.

☐ Changes in stomach size and digestion may mean that your loved one may feel full faster. Too much food heaped on a plate can be overwhelming and confusing. Confronted with a full plate three times per day may actually result in them eating less. Serve smaller meals throughout the day and try plating just one or two foods at a time. They may be more likely to consume more if you offer several small meals and snacks five or six times per day instead.

☐ Don't ask your loved one if they are hungry. They may not remember when the last time was that they ate, that the stomachache they are feeling is actually hunger or that their dry mouth indicates thirst. Asking your loved one whether or not they are hungry may not get you an accurate answer as the concept of hunger or thirst may be difficult to understand at certain stages of the disease process. Questions like "what would you like for lunch" may likewise be too confusing. Try to serve your loved one a small portion of favorite foods and beverages several times throughout the day.

☐ Work to pack as much nutrition as possible into the foods that your loved one is eating. Consuming smaller amounts means that you'll need to be thoughtful in ensuring the calories they do consume are as nutritious as possible. Keep in mind that they still need a balanced diet. Consult your family physician for any caloric guidelines and goals for daily intake of fresh fruits and vegetables, lean proteins, whole grains and low-fat dairy. Try to limit excess sugar, salt and fats that are not only showing to be unhealthful but also may exacerbate certain behaviors associated with Alzheimer's/dementia.

☐ Use contrasting linens and dishes: Changes in depth and visual perception are also a part of the disease process that can make "seeing" food on the plate difficult. Minimize busy patterns and instead opt for a solid colored plate with a contrasting colored place mat to help food items stand out. Keep the table décor simple also. Avoid arrangements of items (like porcelain or plastic fruit) that look edible but aren't.

☐ Finger foods: Decreases in attention span and ability to sit still for long periods of time may prevent your loved one from staying at the table long enough to get the adequate nutritional intake. Try serving finger sandwiches, fruit and veggie slices, cheese and crackers, and other foods that can be consumed away from the table and without having to use silverware.

☐ Keep favorites handy: Your loved one is more likely to eat foods that they enjoy. Help combat decreases in appetite by serving their favorite foods often. That also includes being mindful of the temperature at which you serve meals. Be careful that they are not too hot or cold and reflect your loved one's individual tastes as much as possible. This can help increase enjoyment and percentage of the meal that they consume.

☐ Offer fluids frequently: To decrease the risk of dehydration offer water, juices and higher water content snacks like fruit, popsicles, and Jell-O to supplement water consumption.

☐ Clear liquids can be difficult to see in a clear glass. Adding orange or lemon slices can make it easier for your loved one to identify water in their cup and make it look more appealing. Fluids should be readily available at meal times to aid in digestion.

☐ Prepare the plate: Before serving your loved one, take care to cut up meats and larger food items and add any condiments (spices, gravies or sauces) that they enjoy. Ensure that they have eating utensils available that they are still able to use safely.

- Use adaptive equipment. Consider using scooped plates with higher rims around the perimeter and sectioned plates or bowls to make it easier to get the food out. Large-handled silverware and other devices may help your loved one be more independent with meals and allow for easier, less frustrating dining experiences. "Sippy" cups with lids and foods served in edible containers (pita's, cones, and sandwiches) that can go with your loved one and be consumed on the move are another helpful option for those who can no longer use silverware. Flexi-straws are also an option for liquids.

- Table manners don't matter. Don't worry if elbows are on the table, if your loved one is spilling more than they are actually eating or are chewing with their mouth open. What matters is that they are actually eating. Spills can be cleaned up, and a little ingenuity can make your work post meal a lot easier. Consider a plastic mat like the ones they put under rolling office chairs to put over your carpet underneath their seat to make cleaning the floor a faster job. Use placemats to contain the mess and engage your loved one in decorating their own apron with fabric paint, so they have something more dignified than a bib to wear as a clothing protector while eating.

- Create a routine: Try to offer meals at the same time each day, in the same place and join your loved one at the table. Meal times can be more successful when they are also a social experience and joining with your loved one in partaking of a small meal, or a snack can encourage them to eat. Your loved one may also eat more by "mirroring" you as you offer them visual cues or demonstrate eating yourself.

- Decrease the distractions: Mealtimes can be stimulating enough with all of the sights, sounds, smells, tastes and textures to experience. Be mindful of noise levels and impact of additional stimulation from other people, pets, or media such as television or certain kinds of music. Try to create a quiet, relaxing environment for mealtimes.

☐ Allow twice as much time for meals and then double that. No one likes to feel rushed when they are trying to eat, and your loved one is no exception. If you know that you have an early morning doctor's appointment tomorrow, make a quiche ahead of time that you can just reheat quickly or put together a yogurt and fruit parfait the night before. Spend less time making the breakfast, so your loved one has more time to eat it making things less hectic for you both. Make mealtime an enjoyable experience.

☐ Keep abreast of new studies being conducted that are researching the impact diet and nutrition choices have on overall symptoms, brain health and behavior for persons living with Alzheimer's/dementia. Some of these studies are looking at the things like the impact of brain healthy foods such as walnuts, salmon, and blueberries while other research points to positive results from increasing the consumption of fresh fruits and vegetables while limiting refined sugars for example. There is also much research being done currently to investigate the negative role gluten may play in increasing inflammation in the brain that may worsen the signs of dementia. A simple blood test can determine if your loved one has a gluten sensitivity, identify thyroid problems, high blood sugar or other metabolic anomalies. Ask your primary care physician, dietitian or other medical providers about their specific recommendations regarding your loved one's optimal nutrition.

CHAPTER 8
Managing Medications Made Easier

Persons with Alzheimer's or dementia may react negatively to taking their medications for a variety of different reasons. Caregivers may have to be very inventive to get needed medications successfully administered. Approaches used may need to change based on your loved one's mood, reasons for resisting medication and stage in the disease process. Be patient with the process and know that it's okay to keep trying different approaches. What works today may not work tomorrow. Be flexible.

- ☐ Consider the possibility of any physical reasons why your loved one may be having difficulty taking their medication. For example, are they having an adverse reaction to a medicine? Are they in any pain (poor oral or ill-fitting dentures could be causing mouth pain)? Might they have a sore throat or upset stomach? Have you been noticing any swallowing difficulty? Is the drink temperature you are offering to accompany the pills too hot or cold for sensitive teeth and gums? Alzheimer's can affect the brain's ability to understand and recognize visual input resulting in a problem called Agnosia, which is the loss of ability to recognize people, objects, shapes, smells, and sounds while the sense itself is not defective. They may not recognize their medication, or that they need to swallow it without chewing or even that these are medications that their doctor prescribed for a specific reason.

- ☐ Next, evaluate the environment surrounding medication time for potential distractions or unintended stressors. You might be offering medicines in a place that is potentially upsetting to your loved one. In the bathroom, reflections in the mirror may cause worry. There may be too much noise from a TV or radio, talking adults or noisy children or pets. If you have ruled out physical or environmental factors such as these, there may be other reasons that your loved one is not taking their medication. They may forget how to take medicines that require swallowing without chewing. Sometimes, they may feel like they just took their medication when in reality it's been hours or a whole day between doses.

☐ Provide verbal cues to help coach your loved one through each of the steps involved in taking the medication. In the beginning, simply offering the pills, and watching to make sure that each of the pills is taken. As Alzheimer's and dementia progresses, more support is often required. Try placing the pills in your loved one's hand and giving verbal cues at each step: "It is time to take your medicine. Here is your pill. Put the pill in your mouth. Now take a sip of water. Now swallow the pill."

☐ Provide physical cues as needed by touching or patting the hand that is holding the pill and then touching your loved one's mouth. You could show them by mimicking taking a pill, exactly what it is that you want them to do. Try taking medicines together so they can watch you. If these ideas don't work, try holding the pills to their lips and when they open their mouth, place the pills on your loved one's tongue and then hand them a drink. When holding the pills to his/her mouth no longer cues your loved one to open their mouth, you may have to remind them to open. As your loved one develops problems with swallowing, they may need assistance, such as stroking their throat to promote swallowing.

☐ Offer lots of praise and reassurance throughout. Telling your loved one that they are "doing a great job" or that you are proud of them, that their doctor would be so happy with them. Give them a back rub or hug after taking their pills can do a lot to make medication time more pleasant for you both.

☐ Make medications taking time an unremarkable part of their day. Persons with Alzheimer's/dementia can become suspicious as to why the caregiver is offering medications and may have lost the ability to use logic and reason that can make explaining what they are taking and why, ineffective. Try to avoid announcing that it's "time to take your pills" or "time for your medicine!" Make taking medicines part of their daily routines and fold it into another task when possible, based upon pharmacist instructions (such as take with food versus one hour before eating). Incorporate taking pills into other routines that are less stressful daily activities like, brushing their teeth, having a favorite drink, along with meals, or before bed.

□ Try, try again. If you are met with resistance, come back in a few minutes. Their attitude might be different, or you may try a new approach. Your demeanor can make a big difference. Often your body language and tone of voice will impact your success as a caregiver more than the actual task you are performing or words you are using. Use a big smile, try humming a favorite song and try to appear upbeat and happy.

□ One at a time, or all at once? Discuss the timing with your loved one's doctor to see how you can split up the meds throughout the day, or try taking them together if your loved one would do better with less frequent medication times. Try to offer one or two pills at a time, rather than asking your loved one to take them all at once which might appear overwhelming. Please note, however, some meds should not be taken with others, so do check to see if the medications need to be given with or without food, an hour before a meal, during, or after a meal. Some medications are better absorbed when given on an empty stomach while others need to be given with food to prevent nausea.

□ Use the power of authority. Many seniors are more likely to follow Doctor's orders over well-intentioned family member's advice or pleas. Ask the doctor to give you a "prescription" in writing with your loved one's name on it and phrases such as: "Take your pills! Thank you". Make sure the doctor signs it and go ahead and use this note when needed.

□ Watch carefully and keep a sharp eye out. Some loved ones will hold the pills in their mouths, commonly called "pocketing", and then spit them out after you've stopped watching or left the room. They may not actually be doing that to trick or fight you, however, your loved one may no longer understand that they need to swallow the pill. The delay in swallowing due to their confusion may cause the pill to dissolve in the mouth, and when it starts to taste bad, it then causes them to spit it out.

☐ When all else fails, consider crushing their medicine (if the physician allows) and adding it into something edible. Small amounts of a favorite food especially sweets (jelly, yogurt, applesauce, Jell-O, fruit preserves, smashed bananas, ice cream, pudding or dessert versions of baby foods) can make the medication taste better as well as make medicine time an enjoyable versus stressful occurrence. Some pills can even be dissolved in a warm tea with honey, hot chocolate, smoothie or milkshake.

☐ Try a different formulation. Talk to your pharmacist and ask about "compounding" medications by combining several medications to simplify administering them; they can also check for you to see if your loved one's medications can be given in a cream, chewable version, liquid or another form that they can take easily. The pharmacist may also be able to add flavors to the medications to make them more palatable. If these are not things your pharmacist can assist with, ask them or your health insurance provider for a list of nearby "compounding pharmacies" that specialize in these techniques.

CHAPTER 9
Taking Trips Outside the Home

Trips outside the home can cause increased anxiety due to changes in routine, environment and levels of stimulation. Follow these suggestions to help increase the likelihood of a less stressful experience away from home.

- ☐ Don't rush. Take care to plan out bathing, dressing and meals ahead of time. Getting bathing done the night before and laying out clothes, and printing directions to where you're going will help decrease stress on the day of your outing.

- ☐ When possible call ahead. If you can, call ahead to the places you'll be going (doctor's office, restaurant, pharmacy, store managers, etc.) to let them know that you will be coming in with your loved one and about what time you'll be arriving. In some cases, the staff can assist you in minimizing overstimulation by making their environment a little safer and more comfortable for your loved one when you have given them advance notice.

- ☐ Take someone along. Outings can bring with them unpredictable situations and in these cases it may be helpful to have another pair of hands available to assist you. Don't be afraid to ask friends or family well in advance of your excursion to accompany you.

- ☐ Keep an "on-the-go" bag packed and ready to take with you when you and your loved one are away from home, even for just an hour. Keep snacks, water or juice, extra medications and items of interest when a distraction is needed such as books, photos albums, puzzles, and magazines in your "on-the-go" bag. Also bring a change of clothes for your loved one as well as extra layers of clothing for changes in temperature, additional incontinence supplies and wipes may also come in handy and are better to have and not need than find yourself needing them far from home.

☐ Timing is everything. Choose times of day that fewer people will be where you are going. Planning to be out during "off-peak" times and days when possible, can increase the level of service you experience while decreasing excess noise, stimulation and wait times.

☐ Think about where you NEED to go versus WANT to go with your loved one. Outings can be a lot of work in preparing and planning. As your loved one's disease progresses, outings may become more difficult. Ask family and friends for help with routine errands such as picking up a few items from the grocery store or stopping by the pharmacy to pick up a re-fill. However, meaningful outings can be a very fulfilling part of your loved one's life enrichment even if the goal is just a scenic drive versus an actual destination. When possible, plan for a regular "fun outing" when you and your loved one are up to it.

☐ Outings as activities. Choose destinations that relate to your loved one's past interest or hobbies, centered around easy access foods (cup of coffee, ice cream cone) or provide enough stimulation to keep their attention without being overwhelming. For example, your loved one may no longer show sustained interest for a long enough time period to enjoy a movie, but may like a trip to a park, zoo, museum, aquarium or the like. Places that involve your loved one in some kind type of active participation ("doing") versus just sitting ("watching") may be more enjoyable for you both.

☐ Special safety considerations. Before you go, take into account factors that may affect your loved one's safety while at the location away from home. Pull up a map of the area if possible or call staff to ask about the best route from the car to your destination. Ask about any terrain that may be difficult to navigate including stairs and long hallways, and about nearest restrooms and benches for resting. Ask where would be the best place for you to be seated or wait if there will be long periods of time between arrival and activity.

☐ Keep in communication. Take a cell phone with you for emergencies and let family, friends or neighbors know where you'll be going and how long you expect to be gone.

☐ Have a completed medical history and health information sheet in the car and one on your person at all times while away from home: The Health History Form (sample in Chapter 24) should have your loved one's medications, allergies, diagnosis, medical providers, insurance and emergency contact information noted. Trips outside the home can cause increased anxiety due to changes in routine, environment and levels of stimulation. Follow these suggestions to help increase the likelihood of a less stressful experience away from home.

CHAPTER 10

Family and Friends-
Secrets of Successful Visits

Having company over, even close friends and family, can be a source of potential stress. Follow these suggestions to make interactions more comfortable and enjoyable.

- ☐ Don't isolate. Often caregivers report that one of their biggest sources of sadness is the decreased contact with friends and family as their loved one's signs and symptoms of dementia increase. Resist the urge to limit social interaction as maintaining relationships is healthy for you and can also provide needed socialization for your loved one.

- ☐ Communicate openly. Alzheimer's/dementia are diseases that affect not only the person with the diagnosis but also impact all those that they come in contact with them. You will likely be more comfortable with each other if you can discuss what's happening at home. Preparing visitors and guests about what to expect and any changes they may notice (physically or cognitively) before their arrival can give them time to adjust to the changes that will affect their visit without feeling "put on the spot".

- ☐ Differentiate the disease from the person. Let visitors know that as a result of the disease process, your loved one may say or do things that they normally wouldn't and that they may not fully understand the effect of their words and actions. What visitors see may be more related to the disease, not the person, and they should not take anything personally or be judgmental.

- ☐ Share successes. Share scenarios with visitors to help them feel more at ease with the "to do's" before they get to your home. Feel free to be specific. For example: "Currently, your uncle really enjoys talking about his high school baseball team" or "He has trouble remembering names and dates, so, try to avoid correcting him and try just to listen." The fact that he is talking with you indicates that he enjoys your company even if what he's saying may not be factual or make perfect sense to you. Try to be in the moment and share your loved one's reality and encourage others to do the same by showing them how to communicate without a lot of correcting.

☐ Plan the visit. Think about what time of day your loved one would do better with visitors and guests. Be sure to plan around necessary excursions (doctor appointments etc.) to avoid too much activity or disruption in routine in any given day that can be physically and emotionally taxing for you both. Discuss the length of the visit ahead of time and set expectations around how long your loved one may be up for a visit.

☐ Offer conversation or activity ideas. Set your loved one and guests up for success during their visit by having items on hand that can be used to promote interaction. Reminiscing using old pictures, collectibles and memorabilia can be a fulfilling interaction for all involved. Use items that relate to a familiar hobby of the past that could be organized or sorted and offer your loved one a chance to "work" on a project with their visitor that can help take the pressure off of connecting verbally when having a conversation becomes difficult.

☐ Have a backup plan. Let visitors know that the visit may need to be cut short if certain things occur. Such as; "Just to let you know, if Mom starts to pace or become anxious, we may need to shorten your visit and let her get some rest".

☐ Take advantage of an extra pair of hands and eyes. A trusted visitor may give you the chance to get some tasks accomplished (if you prepare them properly) that would be difficult when you are alone with your loved one. Asking for assistance with watching your loved one will not only help you get more done, but will also give other close friends and family a valuable chance to help someone they care about while feeling useful through the act of being of service and providing assistance.

☐ Schedule visits and put them on your calendar regularly. Planning is important for both you and your guests. Although much of the disease process is unpredictable, spending time together will allow them to connect and enjoy their fellowship during this most difficult journey. Scheduled visits are more likely to occur and go more smoothly than casual open-ended invitations to "drop by".

☐ Plan on imperfection. Things may not go as planned but take pride in the fact that it took courage for you to set aside any worry or fears about what others may think and provide space for your loved one and your family and friends to be together. This is much more important than what was served, what was said or what occurred. Having company over, even close friends and family, can be a source of potential stress. Try some of these suggestions to make interactions more comfortable and enjoyable for everyone.

CHAPTER 11

Understanding Your Loved One's Behaviors

Understanding and dealing with your loved one's "unusual" behaviors may be one of the most stressful parts of being a primary caregiver and when the new "normal" may feel like anything but, consider these tips listed below to help you get through the moment. It's important to remember that the person with dementia is not deliberately being difficult. Your loved one's sense of reality may now be very different than yours, but still very real to them. Changes in your loved one's thought process caused by dementia (including Alzheimer's) may mean that their ability to comprehend consequences and utilize logic and reasoning are negatively impacted. They might not be fully aware of what they are doing or why.

As care partners, we can't change the way the brain impacted by these diseases, but you can offer some understanding and use the helpful techniques in this chapter to change the way we view behaviors and cope with them. Your response to what your loved one is doing or saying can greatly affect the outcome. Things like your body language, tone of voice, pace of the conversation and word choices during difficult times are key tools for care partners coping with an upset or agitated loved one.

The way you choose to react to your loved one can either serve to support them in feeling validated as they process through what they are feeling or conversely escalate their agitation if they feel patronized, ignored or judged for example. All behavior is really at its core, simply another form of communication. We just need to better understand your loved one's unique behavioral "language".

Consider the each episode of behavior in three phases; before, during and after.

- Before: What was happening immediately before the behavior began that might have triggered it (what were the sights, sounds, smells, and stimuli present)?

- During the episode: How did your loved one express themselves (what were they doing and saying?)

- After the behavior: What worked well (and what didn't) while trying to support your loved one at that moment? How did you validate what they were feeling and experiencing? How were you able to help reassure and comfort them? What techniques were ultimately most effective in helping them feel better?

Before: *What was happening immediately before the behavior began that might have triggered it (what were the sights, sounds, smells, and stimuli present)?*

- ☐ Focus on the WHY and not the WHAT. Often, behaviors can communicate an unmet need. Seek first to understand WHY your loved one may be behaving this way rather than WHAT it is that they are actually doing. For example, a person who disrobes may be feeling that their clothing is too tight, too hot or too itchy, or may need to use the toilet.

- ☐ Your loved one's behavior can often be a reaction to stress or a frustrated attempt to communicate. If you can establish why they're stressed or what is triggering the discomfort, you should be able to resolve the problem behavior with greater ease.

- ☐ Are your loved one's needs being met? Could they be tired, need to toilet? Be hungry, thirsty, or in pain? Search for any potentially unmet needs.

- ☐ Does changing their environment or the atmosphere help to comfort the person?

During the episode: *How did your loved one express themselves (what were they doing and saying?)*

- ☐ Validate their feelings. Letting them know you understand that they are upset and you want to help. Try repeating back key words or phrases that they are using to assure them that they've been heard. Tell them "I'm sorry" that this happened, or that they are feeling this way etc. Acknowledge that you understand where they are coming from with phrases like. "I understand" or "You're right". Search for opportunities for agreement, "I would be upset too" to show that you are in this together. Before you can resolve their concerns, you will likely need to give them time and space to vent or express themselves. Introducing a solution too quickly can actually increase agitation.

☐ Let your loved one feel their feelings. Their experiences and emotions around what is causing their behavior is an important part of self-expression. They may not have access to the same range of communication tools that you and I can use freely; it's important to create space for them to share what they can, how they can. Think about a time that you were really upset or hurting emotionally and were venting or sharing those frustrations-how would you feel if someone told you to "just calm down" or "don't worry about it"? Would those types of statements serve to increase or decrease your stress level? As human beings, we all share a need to feel heard, to feel like our feelings and opinions matter and that we have the right to feel the way we feel without relying on another's approval. Just because your loved one has dementia (including Alzheimer's) doesn't mean that they still don't have the same human needs that we do. When we're upset we all still hope for the same things our loved one does; someone to talk to or be near that will listen to us, seek to understand us, empathize with us, care about and comfort us.

☐ Remember, your loved one responds to your facial expression, the tone of your voice, and body language far more than the words you choose. Use eye contact, a smile, or reassuring touch to help convey your message and show your compassion.

☐ Try not to take problem behaviors personally and do your best to maintain your sense of calm. Your loved one may have difficulty expressing how they feel or why and sometimes frustration or fear for example can manifests itself as anger, and often it is directed at whoever happened to be nearby. You may be the recipient of harsh words and angry gestures. I know this is really hard to keep in mind, but try to remember that these outbursts and feelings are part of the disease process, not about how your loved one feels about you, but more about how they feel regarding any given situation.

☐ Be accepting instead of contradicting. Don't correct them; instead look for opportunities to agree. If your loved one is insisting on the keys, instead of saying "No" for example, try "Yes, I'll make sure you get your keys as soon as the mechanic is done with the car. Where should we go first?"

☐ Use a cooling off period if needed, when possible. If safe to do so, give your loved one some space or breathing room. Even if you just sit a little further away from them or watch them from another room, give them a sense of freedom and personal space as they work through their feelings. Sometimes persons with dementia (including Alzheimer's) will need to express themselves physically when they can no longer communicate the way that they want to verbally. Create a safe and supervised space for them to pace (even around the house) or walk around and get outside for a breath of fresh air if possible.

☐ Try to put yourself in their situation. In addition to their words, look at your loved one's body language and try to understand what he or she might be thinking, what they might be feeling or what it is that they are trying to express.

☐ It's OK for your loved one to feel their feelings We aren't always cheerful either and when we are experiencing something upsetting or stressful, we all have every right to get upset. In fact, sometimes when these things happen in our life, we want the fellowship of others, not because we want them to "fix" it, but because we want to know we aren't going through it alone. Sometimes you being there for your loved one is more important than offering a solution.

☐ If you can't fix everything, fix something. There may be reasons that you aren't able to accommodate your loved one's requests, if you can't give them everything they want try giving them at least something that they want.

❑ Consider the "BREATHE" acronym to keep these tips handy when you need to remember these techniques quickly.

Biography 🦋 Based Care®
"BREATHE "Through the Behavior Quick Tips

Before you react or respond, take a moment to BREATHE – remember this handy acronym to help you assess your loved one for any unmet needs that they may want to share with you:

B-   **BED?** Are they tired and in need of rest? Show them a comfortable and quiet place to rest with soothing music, blankets with soft textures and calming smells like lavender.

R-   **RESTROOM?** Does your loved one need to use the toilet? Take them to the bathroom and offer any assistance they may need.

E-   **ENGAGE IN ACTIVITY?** Are they bored and wanting for something to do? Have some activity supplies readily available and on hand. Create space for them to do something with you, ask for their help, focus on what they do well and enjoy.

A-   **ANXIOUS or AFRAID?** Is something causing them distress or upset? Listen to them and validate their feelings if they need to vent. Offer reassuring words and a comforting touch if they seem open to being calmed.

T-   **THIRSTY.** Could they be dehydrated or thirsty? Offer flavored water, juices, popsicles or fruit, or a nice cup of tea or hot chocolate.

H-   **HUNGRY.** Are they ready for a meal or snack? Offer finger foods, a favorite snack or treat and if possible, include them in preparing it or share it with them.

E-   **EXPERIENCING PAIN AND/OR DISCOMFORT?** Take note of any wincing, or favoring of certain areas on the body, changes in mobility/ movement, redness, swelling or other outward signs of physical distress. Be sure to reach out to your physician or healthcare provider to report any signs or symptoms of illness or injury.

After the behavior: *What worked well (and what didn't) while trying to support your loved one at that moment?*

☐ After the moment has passed, and your loved one is calmer, take some time to reflect on what happened start to finish and use each occurrence of behavior as a learning tool to support you in decreasing the frequency of upsetting behaviors for your loved one.

☐ Look, Listen, Learn: Take note of when certain behaviors occur and try to identify what triggers them. Take note of the time of day, the physical environment, the sights, sounds, and smells that were present, even people or pets that may have contributed to your loved one's behavior.

☐ How did you react to the problem behavior? Did your reaction help to calm the situation or did it make the behavior worse?

☐ How did you validate what they were feeling and experiencing? How were you able to help reassure and comfort them? What techniques were ultimately most effective in helping them feel better?

☐ What's not okay? People with Alzheimer's/dementia often exhibit behaviors that are unpredictable and may be outside the bounds of what others consider "normal" or socially acceptable. It may be tough to know when to worry and when to be flexible. In general, try to remember that these behaviors do not define the person, they are a bi-product of the disease and if your loved one had the ability they would probably choose to act differently.

☐ Practice patience and forgiveness. The disease, not the person, is likely causing these things to occur. Try to let things go and avoid holding a grudge over something they may not have meant to do or say, or even remember doing. The exception is if your loved one becomes a physical danger to themselves or others. Physically or mentally abusive behavior is not okay. Even a one-time occurrence should be communicated to your physician or other healthcare/mental health provider immediately to ensure your loved one's safety as well as your own.

On the following page is Biography Based Care's "Dementia (including Alzheimer's) Behavior As Language Worksheet" that helps you communicate with others (family, friends, care providers, physicians, and visitors) what types of behaviors your loved one is engaging in currently and what works best for them in those specific situations.

Biography ❦ Based Care®

Dementia (including Alzheimer's) "Behavior as Language" Worksheet

Understanding and dealing with your loved one's "unusual" behaviors may be one of the most stressful parts of being a primary caregiver. It's important to remember that the person with dementia is not being deliberately difficult. Your loved one's sense of reality may now be very different than yours, but still very real to them. Changes in your loved one's thought process caused by dementia (including Alzheimer's) may mean that their ability to comprehend consequences and utilize logic and reasoning are negatively impacted. They might not be fully aware of what they are doing or why.

All behavior is really at its core, simply another form of communication. We just need to better understand your loved one's unique behavioral "language". The way you choose to react to your loved one can either serve to support them in feeling validated as they process through what they are feeling or conversely escalate their agitation if they feel patronized, ignored or judged for example.

Use the worksheet below to help de-code your loved one's behavioral language. This is great information to share (with family, friends, care providers, physicians, and visitors) with others that interact with your loved one so that they might be better prepared and feel more comfortable with the types of behaviors your loved one is engaging in currently.

Behavior	Before	During	After
For example: pacing, insisting they need to go home, wanting to drive the car or looking for their Mother etc. Be as specific as possible	What was happening immediately before the behavior began that might have triggered it (what were the sights, sounds, smells, and stimuli present)?	How did your loved one express themselves (what were they doing and saying at the time?	What worked well while trying to support your loved one at that moment? What made your loved one feel better? What words or actions might cause negative outcomes and should be avoided next time?

CHAPTER 12

Exit Seeking and Wandering- What You Need to Know NOW!

The Biography Based Care® Reduce the Risk of Wandering tools were created to help reduce the risk of wandering by helping care partners learn more about the potential triggers, interventions and emergency responses required when a loved one has the potential to wander or has wandered.

Each person with dementia (including Alzheimer's) has unique needs and wants and exhibits altered behaviors at different phases in the disease process. Wandering is one of the most dangerous behaviors exhibited because your loved one can become lost or injured. Be prepared for your family member to wander, even if they have never done so before. Do not assume they will not start. In fact, the Alzheimer's Association estimates that as many as 60% of Alzheimer's patients wander away from home. If your loved one is already a regular wanderer, you know from experience that you have to be ever vigilant at all times in protecting their safety.

DISCLAIMER: *It is not possible to eliminate the risk of wandering 100% of the time, but care partners may be able to reduce the incidents and better respond to this risky behavior by having a specific plan in place based on your loved one's individual needs.*

In this chapter, you'll find:

- ✓ Potential Triggers that May Cause Wandering
- ✓ Wandering Intervention Ideas
- ✓ Programs Available to Assist Those that Wander
- ✓ Reduce the Risk of Wandering Home Safety Checklist

✓ Wandering Incident Emergency Response Steps

POTENTIAL TRIGGERS THAT MAY CAUSE WANDERING

Below are some of the most common reasons persons with Alzheimer's /dementia have the urge to exit seek or wander. Knowing the reasons behind this behavior may help you fulfill an unmet need or offer an alternate solution before wandering occurs.

☐ Searching for an item they believe is lost, looking for a specific person, or trying to get to a specific place. Your loved one may not recognize their current surroundings and may be searching for "home" which can refer to an idea or place from their remote memory or familiar past. Where they grew up in their early adult years, for example.

☐ Experiencing delusions. Your loved one may be trying to fulfill a responsibility from their long-ago past, such as going to work or searching for a parent, sibling or child.

☐ Escaping a perceived danger or threat. Your loved one may be frightened by his/her current situation (wanting them to take a bath or medications, get in the car, etc.) or fearful of noise, a strange visitor, or even the belief that someone is trying to hurt them.

☐ Agitation, which is a prevalent symptom of both Alzheimer's/dementia, can manifest itself as a kind of restlessness and can also be brought on by a lack of exercise, change in normal routine, or need for life enrichment activities.

☐ Recent medication change. Alert your loved one's physician if you notice any behavioral changes after medication adjustments.

☐ Is your loved one experiencing any pain or discomfort? Seek to identify any potential physical reasons — too hot or cold, uncomfortable clothing, sitting too long or sitting in the same position, the need to use the bathroom, being hungry or thirsty.

□ Try to determine if your loved one is in pain by conducting a visual assessment to look for bruises, swelling, abrasions or other evidence of physical pain. Gently touch each major body part while asking them "yes" or "no" questions to determine whether or not it hurts.

□ Another technique that aids care partners in identifying areas of pain is to watch for signs that your loved one is favoring an injury. Does it seem as those it hurts to bear weight when they walk or stand? Is your traditionally right-handed loved one using their left hand more, all of the sudden? Is sitting suddenly painful or are shoes starting to hurt? Being in tune with your loved one's body language can serve as an indicator that they are hurting, especially when they are no longer able to communicate those needs verbally.

WANDERING INTERVENTION IDEAS

□ Make sure your loved one's basic needs (might they need to use the toilet, be hungry, thirsty, feel comfortable in their clothing, etc.).

□ Encourage your loved one to walk or exercise with you. Exercise can often help reduce anxiety, agitation, and restlessness. Check with your family physician for appropriate exercise options, and if possible, make their urge to walk a shared activity that you do together in a safe and secure area.

□ Empower your loved one by giving them a sense of purpose and control. Involve them in productive daily activities that may be familiar, such as doing the dishes, folding towels, etc.

□ Create an emergency activity kit with favorite objects, easy "hands on" activity supplies (sorting, crafts, folding, etc.) and calming items like music, books or movies that can alleviate boredom and create a quick distraction. Keep the kit nearby and stocked.

□ Reassure your loved one when feeling lost, abandoned, or disoriented. Remind them that they are loved, and that they are not alone, Share with them who you are, and that they are in a safe place.

☐ Validate their reality to calm agitation and use their motivation to guide them into a different activity. For example, if your loved one is determined to "Get the car right now!" you may want to respond "Sure. But it's not ready yet. They are changing the oil. Let's have a cup of coffee until it's ready." Or, if they are insisting "I need to get to work!" try answering, "You're right! We don't want you to be late. Let's get your face washed and teeth brushed and put on some clean clothes so we can go!" This approach can serve to decrease agitation by using words and actions that seem to be "helping" the person toward their goals vs. correcting or arguing. Once they are in a calmer state, the hope is that it is easier to re-direct them toward a safer activity or different task.

PROGRAMS AVAILABLE TO ASSIST THOSE THAT WANDER

Project Lifesaver (*per www.projectlifesaver.org*)

Project Lifesaver International (PLI) is a non-profit organization whose mission is to provide timely response to save lives and reduce potential injury for adults and children who wander due to Alzheimer's, autism, and other related conditions or disorders.

Per Project Lifesaver International's website, PLI currently has over 1,400 member agencies in 48 states participate in the program—police, sheriff, fire, public safety departments and other emergency responders. The method uses proven radio technology and specially trained search and rescue teams. Citizens enrolled in Project Lifesaver wear a small transmitter on the wrist or ankle that emits an individualized tracking signal. If an enrolled client goes missing, the caregiver notifies their local Project Lifesaver agency, and a trained emergency team responds to the wanderer's area. Most who wander are found within a few miles from home, and search times have been reduced from hours and days to minutes. Recovery times for PLI clients average 30 minutes — 95% less time than for persons without the Project Lifesaver program.

Citizens, municipalities and local Alzheimer's groups have tried to speed the rescue operation by creating registries and "Silver Alert" programs that provide first responders with identification information, physical descriptions and photographs of registrants. While this is a step in the right direction, the identification bracelets worn by the registrants in these programs can only facilitate the rapid return of the individual once they are found. The identification system does not locate the wanderer.

The task of searching for wandering or lost individuals with Alzheimer's, autism, Down's syndrome, dementia or other cognitive conditions is a growing and serious responsibility. Without effective procedures and equipment, searches can involve multiple agencies, hundreds of officers, countless man hours and thousands of dollars. More importantly, because time is of the essence, every minute lost increases the risk of a less than favorable outcome.

If you are interested in enrolling a friend or loved one in the program, visit their website at www.projectlifesaver.org or call them at: 757-546-5502. Project Lifesaver offers two options for families who would like to utilize this life saving, wearable technology:

❑ If your local police, sheriff, fire, public safety departments and other emergency responders already participate in the Project Lifesaver International program (meaning they have the tracking equipment that would "pick up" the signal from your loved one's transmitter and the officers have had special training on this program) then, citizens can contact their local department directly (for a map of agencies in your area that participate, log onto their website at: www. projectlifesaver.org and click on the "Where Are We" tab). Once enrolled in the Project Lifesaver program, your loved one would wear a small water resistant personal transmitter around the wrist or ankle that emits an individualized tracking signal. If an enrolled client goes missing, their care partner notifies their local Project Lifesaver agency, and a trained emergency team responds to the wanderer's area. Each local agency sets the rates for their program and some are even able to offer this service to families for free or on a sliding scale.

❑ If your local law enforcement or public safety agency is not participating in the

Project Lifesaver program, you can request that they contact Project Lifesaver to enroll.

☐ Project Lifesaver's PAL (Protect and Locate) program does not require a local public safety agency to be enrolled in Project Lifesaver. PAL is a program families can access on their own. PAL uses a system that is both a tracking devise and a digital sports watch. PAL is worn on the wrist just like a normal wrist watch. The difference with PAL is that it will protect and locate your "At Risk" loved one if they wander. Along with the digital watch/transmitter PAL also has a portable receiver which notifies the caregiver of a wandering event through the use of GSM & GPS technologies. If an "At Risk" individual wearing a PAL watch/transmitter breaches the PAL perimeter the caregiver customizes (could be your home, your yard, or a small area leading to your mailbox for example) the PAL portable receiver will sound an audible alert and the LCD display will flash red indicating your loved one has wandered from the RF Perimeter you have set. PAL will generate an email alert and send an SMS (text message) with the date and location of the wandering event. For the caregiver's convenience, PAL also has an internet portal available that is accessible worldwide from any PC or smart phone and allows for real time tracking with regular location updates.

If the caregiver presses the "find" button on the portable receiver the PAL watch will determine the location of the individual and the address will be displayed on the portable receiver. If the "at risk" individual wearing the PAL watch/transmitter is lost and chooses to push the panic button on PAL watch the address will be shown on the portable receiver. Both of these events will also update the internet portal and alert emails and/or SMS text message will be sent to the caregiver.

Alzheimer's Association Safe Return Program (*per www.alz.org*)

☐ MedicAlert® + Alzheimer's Association Safe Return® is a 24-hour nationwide emergency response service for individuals with Alzheimer's or a related dementia who wander or have a medical emergency. This program offers

24-hour assistance, no matter when or where the person is reported missing.

The Safe Return Program has a national information and photo database. It operates 24 hours a day, seven days a week, with a toll free crisis line. It works through Alzheimer's Association chapters across the country, law enforcement and other emergency responder agencies.

If an individual with Alzheimer's or a related dementia wanders and becomes lost, caregivers can call the 24-hour emergency response line (1-800-625-3780) to report it. A community support network will be activated, including local Alzheimer Association chapters and law enforcement agencies, to help reunite the person who wandered with the caregiver or a family member. With this service, critical medical information will be provided to emergency responders if needed.

If a citizen or emergency personnel finds the person with dementia, they can call the toll-free number listed on person's MedicAlert + Safe Return ID jewelry. MedicAlert + Safe Return will notify the listed contacts, making sure the person is returned home.

For more information, please contact the Alzheimer's Association by visiting their website: www.alz.org or calling them at 1-800-272-3900.

Project Lifesaver International
Reduce the Risk of Wandering Home Safety Checklist

The Alzheimer's Association® estimates that as many as 60% of Alzheimer's patients wander away from home at some point in the disease process. Even if your loved one has never wandered before, it doesn't mean they won't. Project Lifesaver International™, in conjunction with Mara Botonis, Author of "When Caring Takes Courage" have partnered to provide the community with the "Reduce the Risk of Wandering Home Safety Checklist" It is not possible to completely prevent the risk of wandering. Caregivers are encouraged to consider the steps below to improve home safety.

Use visual cues featuring pictures and words. Persons with Alzheimer's/Dementia often forget where they are, even inside their own home. Visual reminders can provide needed clues and trigger memories. Use photos on the doors to bathroom, and kitchen & "STOP" signs at exits.	Install alarms. There are many wandering prevention alarms on the market that can alert you that your loved one is trying to exit, including sensors and motion detectors. A string of bells placed on/around certain windows and doorknobs can also alert you to their opening.
Provide a safe place to walk and wander within your home or fenced yard for pacing, or exploration. Create a circular route or path by eliminating obstacles and trip hazards (such as high pile rugs, protruding furniture, sharp objects) and inadequate lighting.	Search the many specialty catalogs and websites that feature caregiving products created for Alzheimer's patients, such as motion detectors, electronic beepers, special latches, etc. Use keywords, such as "Alzheimer's Supplies" and Alzheimer's Safety" in your online search.
Use a towel, piece of fabric or cloth (usually fastened with Velcro or rubber band) to "wrap" your door knob to better disguise it and make it harder to turn.	Install safety devices obtained from your local hardware store on all windows, limiting how far the windows can be opened. Place a fence around the house with a lockable gate if possible.
Install wandering-prevention locks such as deadbolts that require a key. Install locks on doors, windows and gates. These locks should require complex maneuvers, thus making it difficult for Alzheimer's/Dementia patients to leave.	In addition to wandering on foot, persons with Alzheimer's or Dementia might attempt to drive. Hide keys to cars and doors out of sight, keep vehicles locked at all times and leave extra keys with trusted neighbors or nearby relatives versus keeping them around your house.
Disguise exits and escape routes. Camouflaging doors and windows can help deter persons with dementia (including Alzheimer's) in their ability to find a way out. Paint doors the same color as walls, or hang curtains on windows that match the color of walls to make exits less visible. Place an end table, bookcase, framed picture or large mural in front of the least used doors or windows.	Create a list of both dangerous and favorite places in your neighborhood that you think your loved one may be. Include such locations as busy crossroads, creeks, bridges, wooded areas, drainage ditches, and/or steep terrain. Include places where your loved one likes to go, or may be trying to get to such as a previous hometown, a local restaurant, shopping center, place of worship, park etc.
Keep a recent photo and detailed physical description of your loved one readily available as well as neighbor phone #' to aid in a search.	Let neighbors know that your loved one may wander. Ask them to notify you if your loved one is unaccompanied outside your comfort zone.

In the Event of Wandering

1. Notify the police. Call 911 or your community's equivalent.

2. If your loved one is enrolled, call Project Lifesaver at: 1-877-580-5433.

3. Let authorities know that you will begin a search of areas in and around your home, yard and neighborhood immediately and will inform them if you find your loved one.

©2015 Mara Botonis, Excerpts from the book, "When Caring Takes Courage"
Produced in cooperation with www.projectlifesaver.org

Biography ❦ Based Care®
Wandering Incident Emergency Response Steps
(Tear this page out and post it where you can find it quickly)

There are a few things you should do immediately to find your loved one as quickly as possible in the event you can't find them and believe they may have wandered. We recommend that you detach and hang this page on the inside of a kitchen cupboard door or the side of the fridge so that it is readily available. In the event you need this information, time will be of the essence, and your quick action may make a significant difference.

1. **Notify the police.** Call 911 or your local Police/Sheriff's department. A missing Alzheimer's patient should ALWAYS be treated as an emergency. Let the authorities know that you'll start a search of the areas in your home, around your yard and neighborhood and that you will inform them if you find your loved one. Give them your cell phone number and keep your cell phone with you with the ringer turned on at all times during the search. In the event that you find your loved one, you can always call the police department and let them know your loved one was found safely. You risk losing valuable time if you search first and call the police later. Many areas have a special "Silver Alert" that issues alerts for missing/at risk seniors that is shared by the media and on local freeway signs alerting a much wider group which can help look out for your loved one. Let the officer know if and when any previous wandering incidents have occurred and where your loved one was located.

2. **Involve neighbors.** Let your neighbors know of your family member's condition and ask them to notify you right away if they see your loved one alone. Give them cards with your phone number on them to keep by their phones. Ask them for their help right away and dividing areas to search in your neighborhood. Remember that the more people you share your loved one's condition and tendency to wander with, the more help you can get in preventing your loved one from getting / remaining lost.

Neighbor Name: _____ Phone: _____

Neighbor Name: _____ Phone: _____

Neighbor Name: _____ Phone: _____

3. **Search.** Look in any potential areas of retreat where your loved one may hide starting with every room in your home and then work from inside out. Move on to look thoroughly in your yard and immediate neighborhood.

4. **Methodically divide up**. Involve others in helping you search areas with a list of both dangerous and favorite places in your neighborhood. Be sure to include busy crossroads, bridges, creeks, overpasses, drainage ditches, or steep terrain. Have a list of places where your loved one likes to go, such as a friend's house, a favorite restaurant, shopping center, house of worship, park, etc.

CHAPTER 13
Preserving Personhood

As you've no doubt already noticed, your loved one's emotional well-being can have a significant impact on their overall physical health and behavior. This chapter focuses on how to improve their quality of life by enhancing whole person well-being for you and your loved one. The "Whole-Person" concept was first presented by the philosopher Mortimer Adler. According to Adler, *"Whole Persons are engaged in a lifetime quest to achieve balance and congruity in all aspects of their lives and continually seek to develop their full human potential."* Organizations, as varied as the US Military, health and human service professionals, teachers and Fortune 500 companies have all used and tailored their application of the whole person concept to help individuals achieve their highest level of fulfillment and success. In this case, the areas of whole person wellness that we seek to enhance are specifically designed for a person with Alzheimer's/dementia.

Biography Based Care's *Living Well with Dementia (including Alzheimer's) Whole Wheel* concept is specifically designed to help you enhance your loved one's quality of life through meaningful, life-enriching activities and interactions. We've divided the whole-person wheel concept into six spoke areas that represent equally important facets of overall well-being. In this chapter, we'll provide a brief overview of each area that we believe is the foundation for making more moments that matter for you and your loved one to share and enjoy.

There is considerable research being conducted around the world to learn more about the possibility that there may be links between therapeutic recreational programs and the decrease in disrupted behaviors and/or delay in the worsening of some symptoms for certain Alzheimer's/dementia patients.

Currently, there is no cure or way to reverse Alzheimer's or dementia, but contributing to the improvement of whole person wellness for your loved one (and yourself) can have benefits beyond measure when it comes to sharing better, brighter days together.

Biography ✻ Based Care®
Living Well with Dementia (including Alzheimer's) Wheel

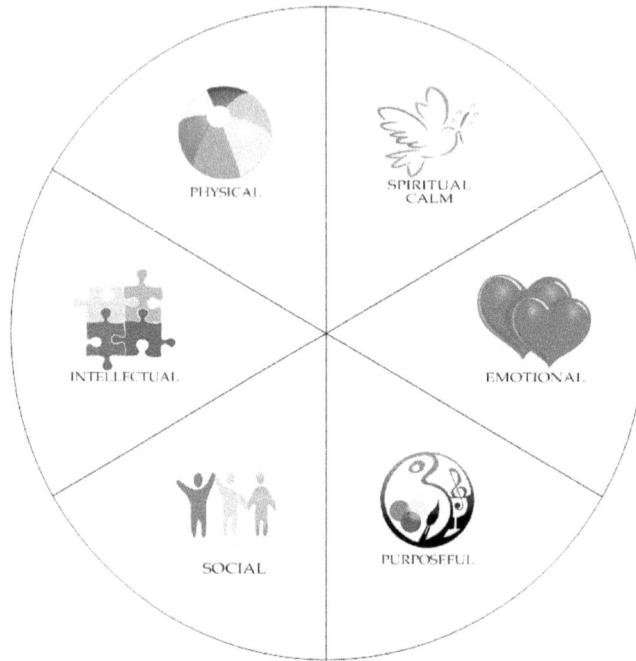

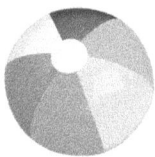

The Physical spoke of the Biography Based Care® Living Well with Dementia (including Alzheimer's) Wheel, from now on referred to as "The Wheel") encompasses many facets of overall physical well-being. These include healthcare-related items (such as proper nutrition, medications, and overall safety, previously discussed as well as activity and interaction-based concepts (such as the power of positive touch and movement) and Alzheimer's and dementia-adapted physical fitness activity ideas for each stage of the disease process. Turn to Chapter 16 for more information on the **Physical** spoke of the wheel.

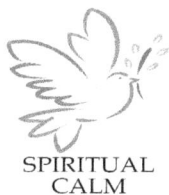

The Spiritual/Calm spoke of the wheel speaks to creating moments of peacefulness, tranquility, or freedom from worry. This spoke is about taking things down a notch when you feel tensions rising. It can assist you in preventing the escalation of certain behaviors. It can help you recognize, appreciate and encourage more peaceful moments together. For some, this is achieved through faith, for others through calming sensory experiences like sounds, sights, and smells. More information on Alzheimer's and dementia-adapted **Spiritual/Calm** activity ideas for each stage of the disease process can be found in Chapter 17.

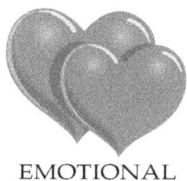

The Emotional spoke of the wheel is about supporting positive feelings (like a sense of belonging, of being loved, feeling safe, or promoting a positive self-image). This can come about in many ways, through reminiscing about something personal and positive, through hands-on activities or communicated through body language and tone of voice. This is about different ways to show your loved one "I love you", "I'm glad we're together", "You're safe here" so that your message may have a better chance of getting through. More information on this spoke and Alzheimer's and dementia-adapted **Emotional** activity ideas for each stage of the disease process can be found in Chapter 18.

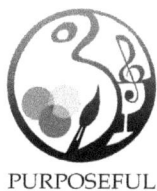

The Sense of Purpose spoke of the wheel is based on a very important part of our Biography Based Care® philosophy. Our passionate belief is that persons with Alzheimer's/dementia are still capable of enjoying a sense of accomplishment and self-worth. Meeting your loved one's need for a sense of purpose can be accomplished by including them in daily tasks that incorporate familiar routines and skill sets that are still accessible to them. Involve them in decision-making and ask for their help whenever possible while setting them up for a successful outcome. This is about helping your loved one feel useful, helpful, that they matter and, more importantly, that they are not a burden. More information on this spoke and Alzheimer's/dementia-adapted **Sense of Purpose** activity ideas for each stage of the disease process can be found in Chapter 19.

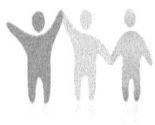

SOCIAL

The Social spoke of the wheel is about how your loved one interacts with other people (including you). It may not mean what it used to before the onset of the disease, but there are still plenty of great ways to connect with your loved one through specific, guided interactions and activities with you, your family and friends. There are still opportunities to connect your loved one to his/her world at large. More information on this spoke and Alzheimer's and dementia-adapted Social activity ideas for each stage of the disease process is found in Chapter 20.

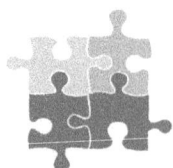

INTELLECTUAL

The Intellectual Engagement spoke of the wheel focuses on creating positive ways to work within your loved one's abilities to stimulate memory and thinking. This is a fun and playful way to connect while gently encouraging your loved one to participate in a wide range of activities. There are lots of choices here, from reminiscing and trivia to simple sorting and easy memory games depending on what stage of the disease process your loved one is going through. The success here lies solely in your loved one's participation. It's all about the "doing" and not the "completing". More information on this spoke and our "failure free" Alzheimer's/dementia-adapted Intellectual Engagement activity ideas for each stage of the disease process is found in Chapter 21.

The Biography Based Care® Alzheimer's/Dementia Whole Person Wellness wheel is meant to give you an overview of the type of psycho-social needs or whole person needs we believe not only persons with Alzheimer's/dementia have a need to fill every day, but that every person does as well.

Think about it for a moment, if you had the power to create your perfect day, if money, time, resources were unlimited; where would you be? What would you be doing? Who would you be joining you? How would you feel?

Before Alzheimer's/dementia entered your life, maybe your perfect day would have been lounging on the deck of an overwater bungalow on the island of Tahiti at sunset with the smells of coconut and gardenia in the air. The sounds of waves caressing sandy shores at regular intervals remind you that you're in paradise, on a day where you are feeling loved, rested and content.

Or maybe you imagined yourself seated at a corner café in Paris eating a warm chocolate croissant after a visit to the Louvre while a light rain falls on a slightly grey day, having taken in centuries of thought-provoking images of the world's most extensive collection of art, while you listen to soft jazz music from the 1940's.

Maybe you're on the shore of a glass calm lake where the morning mist has perfumed the air with the smell of fresh cut grass while you cast your fishing line out in between the calls of the birds singing each other awake and you feel like you have the whole world all to yourself, a secret that Mother Nature saves and shares only with those who are up early enough to appreciate it.

Maybe you thought back to when you towel dried your baby after a bath and thought about the smell of baby shampoo and baby powder and the feel of a warm terry cloth towel and the rhythmic creak of a rocking chair underneath you as you cuddled and held each other before bedtime, knowing right then, at that moment that these nights would pass all too quickly.

A perfect day means something different for everyone.

Chances are, since Alzheimer's/dementia entered your life, your only wish, your best wish, your idea of a perfect day would be to have your loved one "back". To have things "back" to the way they were.

Chances are, your loved one would like nothing more than that as well.

Right now, there doesn't appear to be a way to get there.

But we can help you create another sort of perfect day.

Many experiences don't; require access to long-term memories to enjoy. Despite any deficits created by dementia (including Alzheimer's) you still retain your personhood. Your personhood, your humanness is not dependent on what you know it's about how you feel.

Think about the personhood a newborn baby comes into the world with for a moment. Have you ever seen a baby smile at you when you kiss them or heard them coo with delight when tickle their tiny feet? The way we experience the world around us is present from the moment we enter the world. A baby's person -hood, or their ability to enjoy the examples above don't require them to be able to speak, write, read, or remember. That connection is based on one person connecting with another in a very human way. Open, present, loving and simply showing another that you care. Our loved one's is just like that newborn baby, in that they can still enjoy the warmth of your hug, the feel of sunshine on their face, the sight of your smile and feel of your love. Love doesn't require the brain to remember something it simply feels.

Your loved one may not be able to do things all of the things t

hat the used to before the onset of symptoms, but that doesn't mean that they are can't still experience love, life, and laughter.

The goal is to create the kind of day in which you and your loved one feel like you both matter, like you both belong, that you are safe. A day where you both feel useful, meaningfully engaged, and you are both connected to one another. You can have the kind of day where you are both are having a little bit of fun, a little bit of peace and a whole lot of love.

And that's a pretty perfect kind of day as well.

CHAPTER 14
Finding Time for Fun

The "Ten Minutes Tops Philosophy" is all about making shared activities with your loved one both fun and easy. These activities are easy for you to create and easy for persons with Alzheimer's/dementia to enjoy. Ten minutes speaks to the time you spend preparing these activities and the window of time needed to engage your loved one and capture their attention.

When I think of the ten minutes tops philosophy, I think of it as the difference between a famous chef and an everyday cook. The first, when making a chicken cordon bleu dinner, for example, makes sure to note that she raises her own organic chickens, grows her own organic herbs, and makes her own cheese. I'm not even going to tell you how she comes by the ham that is used in the recipe, cured with honey from the bees she keeps! My point is that this could be the most delicious chicken cordon blue on earth, every bit a symphony of succulence, but who the heck can plan for and grow your own ingredients years, months and weeks before you need them for a recipe? Who has space in their day to spend two and a half hours assembling all the gathered ingredients? If you're like me, the very thought of trying to replicate this tremendous culinary concoction can be so overwhelming that you either go to the freezer aisle for a premade version of the dish that just has to be microwaved, or you make your favorite, easier chicken recipe, add some store bought cheese slices on top with some deli ham, put on some French music and call it dinner!

Sometimes, our idea of perfection, our idea of what it means to "do it right" gets in the way of our even trying at all. Sometimes the ideal version in our heads about creating the perfect day, the perfect activity or "doing things right" based upon what we've read about the stages of the disease and recommended activities has us experiencing more stress than anything else and as a result, some families have articulated that they have had difficulty creating these activities at home. Sometimes the difficulty is because the supplies needed weren't on hand and required a trip to various places for specialty or craft items, or their loved one didn't seem to show any interest in the activity if they did try it, or more often than not, families felt that they simply didn't have the time and energy to "put on" these kind of activities in an already overcrowded day.

In this chapter, we share some general tips about how to make everyday activities more meaningful and enjoyable for both you and your loved one without having to buy, do or finish anything that gets in the way of the primary goal here, which is just to have fun.

- ☐ Everything is an activity. You may want to start be redefining your definition of what an activity is. When we hear the word activities as it relates to Alzheimer's/ dementia, many of us conjure up warm images of smiling seniors merrily crafting or reminiscing over old photos while enjoying a cup of coffee. Well here's the thing, that doesn't always happen. The truth is, almost anything and everything can be considered an activity if it's something that engages your loved one in a safe and positive way for themselves and others. Doing laundry sounds like a chore, and to be honest it is. But, since it needs to get done, the question becomes how can doing the laundry become something that is an enjoyable activity, that involves your loved one, that engages them in feeling successful, needed, useful or loved? What if you asked for their help sorting whites and colors and there is no way they could get it wrong (because you can fix it later)? What if when the laundry was dry, you both took a moment to appreciate the scent of clean linens? What if they helped you match up socks? Or what if you both put on warm pajamas or cuddled under a warm blanket fresh from the dryer? Okay, I know what you're thinking, and no I'm not "nuts." I actually do think there are ways to make laundry fun. Yes, laundry is still a chore that needs to get done, but the idea here is that whatever you are doing can be made more fulfilling if you look for a way to do so. More ideas and examples can be found in Chapter 15: Encouraging Participation in Everyday Activities.

□ Make what you're already doing an adventure. One of the easiest ways to create more meaningful and fun experiences for your loved one is to turn your everyday activities into something exciting. Asking your loved one for help, adding their favorite music or foods can make every day routines something to enjoy versus dread. Think of ways to make tasks into games, outings into adventures and chores into cheerful choices of things that they want to do rather than tasks that you feel you have to accomplish. More ideas on how to do this can be found in part iv of the Appendix: Alzheimer's Adapted Activity Ideas.

□ Be incredibly inclusive. There are few things more heartbreaking for a person with dementia (including Alzheimer's) than being near but not included in the things happening around them. It can feel very isolating to have conversations or actions taking place right in front of you as though you weren't even there. Families who find ways to include their loved one in as many things as possible report feeling less guilt while experiencing more quality time. Even if your loved one can't participate in the conversation or task like they used to, look for ways to make the situation something that they can experience based on their abilities and comprehension. They may not be able to cook dinner with you, but they can fold napkins, or sample the recipes as the official taste tester. They may not be able to fully follow the conversation, but a wink or loving glance from you, sitting next to them or even a simple touch of your hand can let them know that they are important to you, that you're thinking about them. If there is a lot of noise and activities happening, be sure to watch their body language and physical cues of discomfort so you can remedy the situation before feelings are hurt or anxiety increases.

□ Look for ways to build in positive reinforcement. Praise and recognition can make anything better. When one feels like there is no way to do it wrong, fail, or embarrass oneself, you are more likely to try new things or enjoy ones that you may not be as good at as you once were. Creating a space of unconditional acceptance means a better experience for both you and your loved one. If things spill, break, or don't go the way you thought, it's okay. What matters isn't what you DID but how you both FELT. If the cookies you made together burnt or tasted terrible because too much salt was added to the batter, no problem. Focus on the fact that you both loved licking the spoon or eating the dough beforehand, that's a success! Find things along the way to compliment and celebrate. Thank your loved one often for their ideas and contributions.

☐ Find ways to be flexible. Your idea of an activity may be very different than what actually happens. Okay, you've got the puzzle pieces out or have lovingly found a stack of old photo albums, and you're ready to reminisce or play. But... you're the only one that seems to have any interest in that. Instead, your loved one is more interested in staring out the window, picking imaginary lint off of their pants, or looking for their car keys. Go with the flow. Find a way for you to fold into what they are doing or what they are interested in instead of trying to force them to do what you want them to do. If they are staring out the window, put on a nature CD with bird songs, get out a bird book or magazines with pictures of nature. Go for a short walk outside, fill the bird feeder or take them with you to check the mail if weather permits. If they are fussing with clothes, use it as a chance to change outfits or offer a bathroom break. They may be signaling you that they are uncomfortable in their clothing (let's pick out something different to wear), or they have to use the bathroom or that they'd just like to do something with their hands (get something soft out for them to fold and touch). Let them lead you with the cues they are giving based on what they are doing, or saying and learn to use that to support their unmet needs at that moment. That's an activity, and that's okay!

☐ Set about seeing the successes in front of you. The very act of your loved one sitting near you, talking with or looking at you is an indicator that they are interested, engaged and enjoying being with you. What words they use or what they do isn't as important as how they feel. The fact that your loved one wants to interact with you is what really matters. They may not always be able to tell you or show you how they feel about you the way they did in the past, but these moments of little connections with each other are symbolic of a greater love. Being together, being happy no matter what you are doing or saying is a success in itself. Right then and there, that's an out of the park home run!

- If you didn't finish, don't fret. What if your loved one walks off seconds after you start what you're sure was going to be a really fun activity? Or what if they start an activity and a few moments into the interaction they retreat to a place you can't reach them? It's okay. Focus on the time you had that you both felt connected, that they did participate. Make a mental note of what worked. What time of day, or circumstances surrounded the parts of the activity that they liked the best? What did the house sound like, smell like? What things did they show the most interest in and when? If the only part of making cookies together they seem to enjoy is stirring or putting their hands through the dry ingredients, then don't feel like you actually have to bake the cookies. There is nothing wrong with only doing the parts that they enjoy.

- "Shop" the supply store in your house. We all have closets, drawers, attics or garages full of everyday items that can be called into service when it comes to creative ways to engage your loved one. There are many organizations that make a big business out of selling very expensive, pre-packaged special activity supplies for persons with Alzheimer's/dementia that support sorting, reminiscing, and fun in a way that engages your loved one physically and cognitively. However, you don't need a set of colorful wooden blocks, plastic shapes or a special set of books and puzzles to play a game. The truth is, a lot of what you can use to engage your loved one, are items you already have around the house. The added benefit that these items may be familiar on some level to your loved one because they belong to your home and are a part of your shared history only makes it more meaningful.

- Remember your role in making sure things stay fun filled. You are the most significant activity "supply" in this whole process. Your patience, words of encouragement, soothing and supportive tone of voice and loving reassurances throughout whatever activity you choose to do will have a far greater impact on whether or not your loved one has fun than any item you can ever purchase. Your attitude and commitment to making sure that no matter what happens, you'll make sure it retains an air of fun and frivolity is something that doesn't cost any money, but in the end is priceless.

□ Note: Not everything is going to work. Some activities, in fact, might not. So many factors can impact whether an opportunity to engage your loved one was met with any interest on their part. The timing of the activity, their physical and emotional well-being in that moment (fatigue, thirst, hunger, or anxiety level can have a negative impact on them being in the mood to participate). It's okay to have more instances when things didn't go as planned than ones that do, plan on imperfection. Give yourself permission to try new things or modify any activity ideas that you read or hear about to best meet your loved one's needs and capitalize on their interests and abilities.

□ Do be resilient, don't stop trying! Something that was a huge hit with your loved one last time might register a disinterested glance the next time you try it. That's okay. Don't give up; keep looking for a different approach, different ideas, and different ways of offering a variety of activities until you hit upon the combination that works well at that moment. Even if it only worked well for your loved one once and never again, it was still a success!

Life is a series of these small victories, these shared experiences that connect you both despite the disease. Cherish the times when you laughed, played, shared in something that reminded you of a time before Alzheimer's. Enjoy any experience where even for only a brief breath of time you were in touch with the life that was lived long before you knew what dementia was. Accumulating more and more moments that matter along the way, is more important now than ever before. Every one of these moments is a precious gift to be nurtured, protected and celebrated.

In chapter 22, we'll talk about how to make more of these moments every day, how to encourage your loved one's participation, their involvement, in the life that is happening all around them. Creating more moments that matter is one of the most worthy ways to spend your shared days. These moments can be the best salve for an aching heart affected by this devastating disease.

CHAPTER 15

Encouraging Participation in Everyday Activities

As you probably know all too well, a person with Alzheimer's or other dementia may need extra help, time, and support to remain engaged in everyday activities. There isn't an easy answer or fool proof solution for how to keep your loved one connected to their surroundings or the people in their life. However, there are ways for you to encourage their participation in events and activities happening around them. As the disease progresses, you may need to make adjustments to the activity or task to best engage your loved one. Numerous families have shared the following useful tips:

☐ Keep your loved one's skills and abilities in mind. Find activities that build on their remaining skills and talents. A professional accountant might become frustrated over their inability to recognize money, but an amateur might enjoy sorting coins. Be aware of physical limitations. Does he or she get tired quickly or have difficulty seeing, hearing or performing simple movements? By assessing your loved one's skill level, you can better modify the way that you are asking them to participate so that success is assured. Can they sort objects by size or color? Can they button shirts and zip up jackets? Can they follow written commands? Modify activities to make them more or less challenging to fit the skill level of your loved one and find ways to incorporate what they can still do as often as possible. Activities that help the individual feel like a valued part of the household, such as folding towels, setting the table or watering the houseplants can provide a sense of success and accomplishment.

- Pay special attention to what the person enjoys. As we discussed in the previous chapter, you will want to look for favorites. Maybe your loved one always enjoyed drinking coffee and reading the newspaper, for example. These activities may still be enjoyable on some level. Even if he or she is not able to completely understand what the newspaper says, the act of feeling the paper in their hands, looking at the pictures and smelling the aroma of freshly brewed coffee may evoke positive feelings. Repeat favorite activities, and establish a routine. While doing familiar activities, such as sorting objects, or "reading" the paper, keep the procedures the same, but try different content from day to day to keep it fresh for your loved one and you.

- Take note when the person seems happy, anxious, distracted or irritable. If you notice a person's attention span waning or frustration level increasing, it's likely time to end or modify the activity. That goes back to our "10 Minutes Top's philosophy in Chapter 14, if your loved one isn't showing any interest in the first 10 minutes of the activity, it's time to offer a new one. Likewise, look for activities and tasks that can be broken into 10-minute blocks of time to avoid creating frustration or boredom. Let your loved one's behavior be your guide, if they want to continue with something, great! The activity or task shouldn't depend on time or actual completion. Look for things that are okay to leave undone.

- Consider the time of day. Caregivers may find they have more success with certain activities at specific times of the day, such as bathing and dressing in the morning. If something isn't working, it may just be the wrong time of day or the activity may be too complicated. Try again later, or adapt the activity. Select the best time of day for your loved one and offer options. Does your loved one have more energy in the morning, if so, then set outings and appointments for early or mid-day. Is he or she more agitated in the afternoon? Plan on having engaging tasks ready to offer several times per day depending on their mood and interest.

- Help get the activity started. Most people with dementia still have the energy and desire to do things but may lack the ability to self-initiate enjoyable experiences. They may need your help to organize, plan, and complete the task. Put out the things that they'll need either one at a time, or in sequential order. Offer support and supervision. You may need to show your loved one how to perform the activity and provide simple, easy-to-follow steps. Let them watch you do one thing at a time. Put your brush in water, then in the non-toxic paint, then on the paper. Narrate step by step as you go for those that respond better to verbal cues.

☐ Assist with difficult parts of the task. You may need to show the person how to perform the activity and provide simple, easy-to-follow steps. Keep activities very simple and tailored to their current level of ability. The goal here is to create some fun not frustration. Too many decisions may frustrate people with dementia (including Alzheimer's.)

☐ Keep over-stimulation to a minimum. Give both verbal and visual instruction. Feel free to tell how and to show how. If your loved one is accepting, even guide his or her arms and hands gently as you instruct. As the disease progresses, you may want to introduce more repetitive tasks. Be prepared for the person to eventually take a less active role in activities.

☐ Create meaningful activities. This is not about filling your loved one's day with "busy work." Try for activities that your loved one used to do and enjoy. Play up past interests. People with dementia (including Alzheimer's) often maintain old habits and long-term abilities. Try incorporating these retained skills or interests into smaller and more manageable components. Create games based on their interests. Relate to past work life. A former office worker might enjoy activities that involve organizing, like putting coins in a holder or making a to-do list. A farmer or gardener may take pleasure in working in the yard or arranging flowers you've cut, or watering plants.

☐ Include activities that allow your loved one a chance for self-expression. These types of activities could include singing, painting, drawing, music or conversation. Look for ways for them to drive the activity whenever possible. Let your loved one show and tell you what they need to communicate in a variety of ways.

☐ Do activities that let your loved one manipulate materials or work with their hands. Persons with Alzheimer's/dementia still very much enjoy the sense of touch so working with different textures is often an accessible experience far into the disease process.

☐ Don't criticize or correct your loved one. Look for the positive. If your loved one is enjoying a harmless activity, even if it seems insignificant or meaningless to you, encourage them to continue. Offer words of encouragement and positive reinforcement. If your loved one is involved and happy, don't correct them. The goal is to engage the person with Alzheimer's/dementia and encourage in them a sense of success.

☐ Create a positive activity incorporating your loved one's behavior. If your loved one is pacing, offer to take them for a walk. If they are tearing a paper napkin into pieces, get out a magazine for collages. If his or her hand is moving back and forth across your table, provide a cloth and encourage the person to wipe the table. Or, if the person is moving his or her feet on the floor, play some music so the person can dance or tap to the beat.

☐ Keep the work area safe. Be mindful of small items that may present a swallowing risk or non-edible items that look like food. Work with unbreakable plastics. Keep surfaces clean, uncluttered and well lit. Be thoughtful about ensuring their safety in advance of asking them to help or contribute.

CHAPTER 16

Alzheimer's Adapted Activity Ideas: Physical

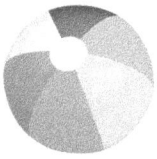

PHYSICAL

As you remember, the Physical spoke of The Wheel encompasses many facets of overall physical well-being. These include healthcare-related items (such as proper nutrition, medications, and overall safety, previously discussed as well as activity and interaction-based concepts (such as the power of positive touch and movement) and Alzheimer's and dementia-adapted physical fitness activity ideas for each stage of the disease process.

Leading a physically active lifestyle can have a very positive impact on overall well-being. Exercise is beneficial for both physical and mental health and can improve the quality of life for people in all stages of dementia. Physical activities can range from simply walking across the room, gentle stretches while sitting, walks or even more active endeavors such as Tai Chi, senior yoga or dancing.

Benefits of exercise and physical activity may include, but are not limited to:

- ✓ Potentially improving overall heart health in general.
- ✓ Opportunities to enhance physical function. Maintaining muscle strength and joint flexibility can also be a way to help your loved one maintain their independence for a longer period.
- ✓ Helping to keep bones strong and dense, reducing the risk of osteoporosis or fractures.
- ✓ Possibly improving cognition - recent studies have shown that regular exercise may improve memory and slow down mental decline for some people.
- ✓ Improving sleep.

✓ Creating opportunities for social interaction which helps reduce feelings of isolation

✓ Potentially help reduce the risk of falls for some persons with dementia as physical activity can improve strength and balance, and help to counteract the fear of falling.

✓ Promoting an enhanced feeling of self-confidence about the body and its capabilities - through improved body image and a sense of achievement.

Here are some things to think about when beginning a physical fitness program for your loved one:

☐ Involve the senses: Take note of which sense(s) your loved one seems to prefer by noting what they do or say, e.g. do they really enjoy the smell of flowers? The taste of a favorite meal? The sound of the birds? Incorporate more activities that call for the use of the sense(s) your loved one seems to experience most successfully.

☐ Consider your loved one's abilities, needs and preferences: Some people will have participated in regular exercise over the years, and the concept will not be new, while others might have exercised very little.

☐ If your loved one has not taken part in any formal exercise for some time or has any health issues, seek medical advice from your family physician or medical provider before commencing any new physical activity.

☐ Be especially certain to obtain any specific guidelines or restrictions on the level of physical activity your loved one can participate in from their primary care physician.

☐ Ask their physician about any special considerations related to these health concerns if applicable:

  -heart problems

-high blood pressure

-unexplained chest pain

-dizziness or fainting

-bone or joint problems

-breathing problems

-balance problems

-frequent or history of falls

These health conditions might not prevent your loved one from participating in an exercise program, but checking with your primary care physician before you get started is recommended.

☐ It is important to choose activities that are both medically appropriate and enjoyable for your loved one based on their unique personal history. Use the Biography tool found in Chapter: 2 to help you identify familiar pastimes or favorite hobbies that can be used to encourage participation.

☐ Exercise can be done on a one-to-one basis or in a small group. Your loved one may like to try a few different activities to see what suits them best.

☐ Know when to say when. If you notice your loved one appears fatigued or exhibits pain or discomfort in any way, STOP!

☐ Hydrate often while enjoying physical activities and make sure to take plenty of rest breaks along the way.

☐ The restorative power of rest cannot be overstated. People aren't designed to be in motion at all times and a person with dementia is no different. Sometimes the unmet physical need is simply for some quiet time and a cozy place with a warm blanket and soft lighting to take a nap or just sit quietly.

Exercising for Alzheimer's/dementia in Early to Mid-stages of Dementia (including Alzheimer's):

During the earlier stages of dementia, there many options for physical activity. Often your local adult day care or family center will offer classes designed for aging participants.

- Seated exercises, music, and dance, tai chi, yoga, as well as swimming are some of the popular forms of exercises you can use.

- Walking – Walking is an ideal exercise for almost all levels of physical ability. You vary the length and distance of your walking route based your loved one's level of interest, enjoyment and level of fitness.

- Gardening – When gardening, your loved one gets the opportunity to be physically active while getting plenty of fresh air. Match their activities with their physical abilities (in later stages try indoor countertop gardens) and create purpose driven physical activities such as raking leaves, watering the plants, weeding, or general tidying.

- Seated Exercises – Seated exercises like marching, making a motion as if riding an imaginary bicycle, raising the arms or legs, and simple stretches create an easy way for your loved one to get a little exercise without increasing the risk of falling or requiring good balance.

- Safer Versions of Familiar Sports - In the early stages of the disease process when motor skills are more intact, your loved one may enjoy Nerf or plastic versions of familiar favorites such as bowling, badminton, tennis, croquet, playing catch or bean bag toss. Video Game versions of many of these games are available and potentially safer and easier to enjoy indoors.

Exercising for Later Stages of Dementia (including Alzheimer's)

Some type of physical activity is still very helpful for loved ones in the later stages of dementia. Gentle and appropriate exercise or stretching can help in reducing the need a higher level of care and delay the use of adaptive equipment (such as walkers, wheelchairs, commode, etc.) by helping your loved one maintain strength and muscle tone. Even walking from room to room inside your house or rising from sitting to standing can have a positive impact.

The following exercises may be beneficial in the later stages of dementia (including Alzheimer's):

☐ Demonstrate how to balance your body in a standing position with your loved one. If necessary, have them hold onto a sturdy piece of furniture for support. Their balance and posture can improve with this exercise, making it easier to complete daily activities like showering or walking to the toilet. Make sure they perform this exercise only when someone else is present, as there may be a risk of falling.

☐ Have your loved one lie perfectly flat on the bed for at least 10-15 minutes every day. This activity will help them stretch their muscles and reduce anxiety. Put on a CD with nature or soothing sounds to help promote relaxation.

☐ Have your loved one sit without any support for a few minutes every day, sitting up as straight as possible. Again, you may have to do this activity with them so they can watch you demonstrate. This activity can help strengthening the muscles in their stomach and back, helping them improve their posture. Make sure they perform this exercise only when someone else is present, as there may be a risk of falling.

☐ Have your loved one simply stand up and move around the house on a regular basis. This activity will help in maintaining strength and balance even as mobility may be decreasing. Please check with your medical provider about whether or not this is appropriate for your loved one.

☐ Small Circles. While your loved one is lying down, gently guide them in making small circles clockwise and then counterclockwise with each hand and foot one at a time to help promote circulation.

☐ As the disease progresses, your loved one may need reminders and some encouragement to move around. Look for ways to encourage activity as tolerated several times throughout the day in small intervals to reduce fatigue.

CHAPTER 17

Alzheimer's Adapted Activity Ideas: Spiritual or Calming

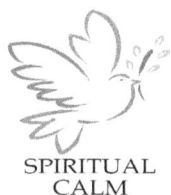

As you recall, the Spiritual/Calm spoke of The Wheel speaks to creating moments of peacefulness, tranquility, and freedom from worry. This spoke is about taking things down a notch when you feel tensions rising. It can assist you in potentially preventing the escalation of certain behaviors. It can help you recognize, appreciate and encourage more peaceful moments together. For some this achieved through faith, for others through calming sensory experiences like sounds, sights and smells work best.

Here are some quick tips for creating a sense of calm with aromatherapy, art therapy, massage therapy, music therapy, and pet therapy, spiritually themed activities and sound therapy.

Aromatherapy: Some essential oils are said to promote calming. These aromas can be found now in most stores incorporated into everything from organic oils to shampoos, candles, diffusers, and soaps. Before using aromatherapy, be sure to make sure that your loved one is not sensitive or allergic. Aromatics that show promise for treating symptoms of Alzheimer's or dementia include:

- Lavender – Is one of the essentials most used in studies of the effects of aromatherapy on those with Alzheimer's/dementia. It is thought to be a calming scent that can be used both at nighttime to help encourage sleep or during the daytime to promote a better mood.

- Lemon Balm –Another essential oil that has been used in aromatherapy for persons living with dementia (including Alzheimer's). Lemon Balm is thought to promote calm and encourage a relaxed mood.

☐ Peppermint –Used to both stimulate the mind and calm the nerves. It is said to help rectify absent-mindedness. Use it in the morning to energize your loved one and stimulate appetite.

☐ Bergamot – Mood elevating, calming, and balancing. Bergamot is believed to reduce stress, anxiety, and mild depression.

☐ Palmarosa - with its sweet hint of floral, yellow color and water like viscosity is quickly gaining favor as users report feeling an uplifting or calming of the mind.

Art Therapy

Both viewing and creating works of art can be therapeutic. Interpreting and creating art, after all, is up to the individual, there's also the freedom of expression. Working on an art project can also help release emotions in a safe, healthy way. Working in a material with their hands is a great way to shift the focus from anxiety to creativity.

☐ Don't worry if your loved one wasn't very artistic in the past, there is no right or wrong way to express themselves. You can support your loved one in working with the colored pencils/paints and paper by letting them know that they do not have to draw anything specific. You can let them just create whatever comes to mind or have some old greeting cards, calendars with pictures or magazines handy for inspiration.

☐ Provide safe, non-toxic, easy-to-use materials and encourage your loved one to spend time with them. There are lots of wonderful websites that offer free adult coloring pages in many themes. If you're unsure how to get started with an art therapy experience with your loved one at home, look into adult day care programs in your area that offer art classes. Find out more about bringing your loved one to their art events or getting started on your own.

☐ Viewing familiar or favorite works of art can transport your loved one to a calmer, happier times. Have these images on hand in coffee table books or hanging on your wall. Engage your loved one in conversation by asking questions and pointing out interesting features. For example, a famous Norman Rockwell illustration entitled "Freedom from Want" with a family gathered around a holiday turkey can evoke many pleasant memories and opportunities to talk about family, food and the holidays.

Massage Therapy

When we think of massage therapy, we likely imagine a spa with professionally trained masseuses. While in the early stages of the disease process, your loved one might enjoy that, you can also the healing power of touch yourself right at home. Touch can trigger the relaxation response, lower blood pressure, and in some cases, even reduce the pain of chronic diseases. Massage is also thought to help people with chronic diseases in sleeping better, decreasing their pain level and improving mood.

☐ To try this at home, ask your loved one if it's okay to put lotion on their hands or give them a gentle backrub. Seek permission first and ensure that you let your loved one know in advance where you'll be touching them (hand, back) and what you'll be doing ("I'm going to put some lotion on your hands now, Mom") to decrease fear and uncertainty.

☐ Someone who's apprehensive or has never had a massage may want to start with hand, foot, or back rubs. Let your loved one guide you. Look for visible clues for feedback—does your loved one appear relaxed or uncomfortable? Adjust accordingly.

☐ Massage therapy only works when the person feels at ease with it. If your loved one is very sensitive to touch or may feel uncomfortable with even a family member touching him or her in this way, then don't continue.

☐ You don't have to ask your loved one to undress, lay face down on a massage table at a salon with a professional practitioner that they don't know to harness the benefits of the power of touch. Hugging, holding hands, touching your loved one gently on the arm, leg or back when you are talking with them are all good examples of how to incorporate the therapeutic power of touch.

Music Therapy

Have you ever found yourself absentmindedly singing a song you haven't heard since high school and all of a sudden you are surprised to realize that you know all of the song lyrics. That's the power of something we dementia care professionals call "musical memory". Your loved one might not be able to remember what they had for lunch or be able to recognize family and friends, but when a song from decades ago plays, they can sing along with the lyrics. Listening to familiar music can be a wonderfully uplifting experience that can help improve your loved one's mood and offer another way for them to express themselves and connect with others. Often called the universal language, music allows people from varied backgrounds to find commonality through their shared enjoyment of particular songs and genres. The same is true for Alzheimer's patients as they still may remember a preference for a particular genre of music.

□ Prompt your loved one to reminisce about their past and interact with you about the places and times that their favorite songs represent.

□ Pick music that's familiar to your loved one if you have an idea of which artists and songs they like. When in doubt, try music from movies and radio that were popular during the decades that they were in their 20's, 30's and 40's. You can also try instrumental music that offers a soothing background.

□ Some people with dementia (including Alzheimer's) enjoy feeling a part of the rhythmic sounds they are hearing and even if they have never played an instrument, might start clapping their hands or tapping their feet along with the beat. You can also look for lap piano, small drum, hand bells, maracas, tambourines, or xylophones that can simply be shaken, strummed or plucked without any pressure to play a specific piece of music or follow the notes.

Pet Therapy

Many pet owners will attest there is just something soothing about the love of an animal. Even just seeing or having a pet nearby can markedly improve mood and ease depression. In this kind of therapy, the animal -- whether it's a bird, dog, cat, fish tank, or other pet(s), these creatures can be the center of some very meaningful moments at any stage of the disease because these human-animal interactions can stimulate verbal communication without requiring it to be a beneficial experience.

- ☐ If you already have an animal at home, be sure to support interactions that are positive for both the pet and your loved one. Making sure the animal is in the mood to cuddle or play is as important as making sure your loved feels this way also to avoid potential injury or discomfort.

- ☐ Ensure that your pet is up to date on all immunizations and has well-groomed nails or claws to reduce the risk of injury.

- ☐ Guide your loved one with simple verbal instructions or demonstrate the interaction to help them get started. Gently place the animal near your loved one (if okay with both!) and model gentle petting or ask for your loved one's help in filling food and water bowls.

- ☐ No pet of your own? No problem! Bird-watching or looking at an aquarium seems to have just as positive of an effect. Try setting up an aquarium or placing bird feeders outside a favorite window.

- ☐ Nature DVD's featuring aquarium or birds scenes. Pastures with horses or kittens and puppies playing can also provide some benefit. Pick visuals that feature their favorite animals for the best results.

- ☐ Stuffed animals in the shape of a favorite type of animal or even a specific breed can also be a great substitute for the real thing if your loved one is no longer able to take care of or be with a long gone beloved family pet.

Spiritual Activities

Whether your loved one's spiritual activities include prayer, religious services, or visits with someone who offers faith-based counsel, spiritually themed activities can have a very positive and calming effect on many persons living with dementia (including Alzheimer's). Activities that incorporate spirituality and faith based opportunities offer stress relief, hope, and reassurance. What's more, religious participation usually gives your loved one a chance to socialize and participate in time-honored traditions from their past in a way that they find accessible in the present.

☐ Arrange for your loved one to continue attending their routine religious services as long as possible. If their behavior is erratic and sometimes disruptive, see if a "quiet room" is available for private reflection. Also, consider going during off-peak hours and days to decrease the risk that the environment may be over-stimulating with too much noise or large crowds.

☐ Ask for a home visit. Many churches and spiritual organizations have formal home visit programs to bring faith-based fellowship to those that are homebound. Check your local church or yellow pages for more information. Be sure to be mindful about who you invite into your home and ask about the process to train and check out these volunteers that the organization uses before you have someone you don't know over. If in doubt, check it out.

☐ Find an old hymnal or songbook or CD with faith songs dating to your loved one's youth, they might enjoy it more at home than newer editions. Try singing them to your loved one if they can't sing themselves.

☐ Consider reading aloud from the Bible, or other familiar religious texts or inspirational short stories if your loved one responds well to this.

☐ Be creative in identifying things that may nourish your loved one's spirituality, in a less traditional way. For some people, that's a walk in the woods, looking up at the night sky, listening to classical music, or meditation.

Sound Therapy

☐ Different than music with recognizable words and melodies, sound therapy refers to the positive effects of certain noises. Knowing your loved one well can help you identify which sounds may best create a positive reaction.

☐ Use the biography form in Chapter 2 to look for your loved one's familiar places, people and times in their life to create a soundscape that best suits them. For example, did your loved one like the beach vacations you would take together as a family? Try ocean or birds sounds to remind them of those happy times and places.

☐ Have a CD on hand with the sounds of the wind, ocean, birds chirping or tropical rainforest sounds to create a pleasant environment.

☐ Think of other pleasant sounds such as children laughing or playing, sounds of a train or sailboat. Soundscapes can be made by downloading these custom noises from the internet or looking for themed CD's or TV shows that incorporate these. When possible, enjoying these sounds in person.

CHAPTER 18

Alzheimer's Adapted Activity Ideas: Supporting Emotional Needs

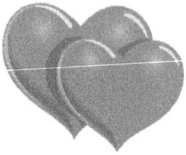

EMOTIONAL

The Emotional spoke of The Wheel is about supporting positive feelings (like a sense of belonging, of being loved, feeling safe, or promoting a positive self-image). This can come about in many ways, through reminiscing about something personal and positive, through hands-on activities or communicated through body language and tone of voice. This is about different ways to show your loved one "I love you", "I'm glad we're together", "You're safe here" so that your message may have a better chance of getting through.

Much of Alzheimer's/dementia care in the past has focused on trying to manage the physical needs of the disease (medications, toileting, bathing, dining, etc.) while perhaps minimizing the emotional ones. A lack of attention to emotional needs can make a patient more introverted, withdrawn and even increase anxiety or negative behavior.

Here are several ways to engage with a person with Alzheimer's/dementia differently, focusing on the emotional needs to uplift their spirit and soul.

Throughout the disease process, continue trying to communicate with your loved one. As we discussed in Chapter 3, there are lots of different communication methods you can utilize, the important thing is to continue trying to keep them engaged, so they don't feel ignored or left out.

Focus on feelings, not facts. Look for ways to draw out what the heart remembers, even if the mind forgets. Certain emotions are attached to different memories. Even when your loved one forgets something, they still know the feeling of that recollection. The result is that even if your loved one forgets a conversation they had with you, there is still a benefit. Subconsciously a person with Alzheimer's / dementia may remember and feel the positive attitude from talking to you even though it is a forgotten experience. Your loved one may not remember the name of a familiar relative in an old photo, but they may still smile when they see that face.

Remember what they can still do, what they do have. While they may be losing their ability to remember or handle everyday tasks, the ability to experience emotions, will always remain at some level. Often the cause of negative behavior starts with hurt feelings. When you focus on fulfilling their emotional needs supporting their feelings of being loved, valued, purposeful and safe for example, you will likely see very positive improvements in your relationship with your loved one and their behavior.

- ☐ When it comes to your affection for your loved one, find ways to say it and show it frequently. Identify and use their preferred sense to increase the chances that your message of love will "get through". If your loved one responds better verbally, tell them how much you care about them. If they seem to appreciate a nice back rub or hug, then try to make more time for these things. Do you have a loved one who appreciates ice cream or a favorite meal? A great way to show them you care is incorporating favorite songs, sights, music, photos or movies. The more ways you can show your loved one that you love and appreciate them, the more likely they will be to get the message.

- ☐ Manage your own stress level. At times caring for your loved one can take its toll on you causing frustration and fatigue. Person's with Alzheimer's/dementia are still very able to pick up on your stress level as your body language, word choice, and tone of voice changes have a big impact on their emotional well-being. Be mindful of your own emotional wellness and seek ways to take a "time out" when you might need to calm down or decompress for a few moments before re-engaging your loved one.

□ Focus on your loved one, not on their disease. Take care to treat them like a person not a patient. Not everything ends when the memory begins to fade. Even though Alzheimer's disease takes a lot away from our loved ones, there are still many parts of their personhood that remain intact. Focusing on your loved one rather than the disease allows for your relationship to have hope for the future. Dementia (including Alzheimer's) can't rob a person of everything he or she feels and is.

□ As we stated in previous chapters, all behavior is communication. Look beyond the illogical behavior to the root cause. A person with dementia (including Alzheimer's) does what is logical in their mind though it seems like strange behavior to everyone else. They may pace to counteract boredom or make sounds to show that they need something. Trying to interpret the meaning of the behavior and engaging with your loved one will be much more successful and beneficial than simply ignoring them.

□ Allow your loved one to make small decisions, even though they might struggle with tasks. Someone with dementia may not be able to do or decide certain things for themselves, but allowing them to make little decisions will do a world of good. The simple task of choosing what to wear or whether they want some jam on their toast, for example, helps to keep certain cognitive abilities intact.

□ Assist family and visitors in evaluating and promoting comfort strategies as you find which ones work best for you loved one. Preparing others for what they might expect when with your loved one and how you'd like them to behave (reassuring, patient, positive) can help these interactions go more smoothly. More information on successful visits with others can be found in Chapter 10.

□ Encourage your loved one to continue using abilities, e.g., hold a cup/spoon/brush, sit up to eat at table or tray, walk, exercise extremities, hum or sing, etc. Allow plenty of time for them to accomplish these tasks at their own pace and then use the opportunity to foster an improved sense of self-esteem by praising their success.

◻ Take steps to decrease fear and uncertainty whenever possible. Give verbal reassurances often by saying things such as "You're doing great!" or "I'm glad you're here with me", or "You're in the right place". Take care to avoid startling your loved one by standing in front of them when speaking. Stay in their line of sight before touching, stand beside them before pushing the wheelchair, tell the person where you are/what you're doing whenever you are out of their line of sight, etc. Remind them of who you are and what you'll be doing before you do it. "Mom, it's me, Mara and I'm going to brush your hair now". If your loved one no longer relates to their relational role with you (i.e. she no longer responds to "Grandma"), it's okay to use their first name or nickname. It's all about creating trust through familiarity.

◻ Therapeutic lying. Some recent media reports have discussed the idea of 'therapeutic lying'. This is where someone may lie to a person with dementia as it may be more beneficial for them than knowing or being reminded of the truth. For example, it could be that a person with Alzheimer's/dementia is asking to see an old relative who is no longer alive, and someone caring for them may consider lying to them in response to help keep them calm or happy. There are a number of ways to handle this difficult situation and the better you know your loved one, the less complex this is to deal with. It's important to consider that lying to a person with dementia – for example telling them that their relative will be back soon – would only provide a temporary solution and could exasperate the situation later on. Equally, telling the truth could cause that person significant distress. Distracting them could also leave the person more confused and frustrated.

Another possible response is to validate their feelings. By telling them that you understand their emotions and why they are asking for that relative, you can help them to feel supported and secure. For example, "I understand you miss Bill, I do too. I like his kind blue eyes and how he likes to go fishing. Did you ever go fishing with him?" Engage in reminiscing about positives related to the situation to take away the hurt of not having access to that person or place any longer.

❑ In this circumstance, to begin to understand what a person living with dementia might be saying, first try to consider the context of the question being asked. Look beyond what the person is saying to try to find the meaning behind the words, and respond to the feelings they may be expressing without getting caught up in whether what they are saying is correct. Listen with your heart not your head.

CHAPTER 19

Alzheimer's Adapted Activity Ideas: Promoting a Sense of Purpose

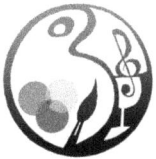

PURPOSEFUL The Sense of Purpose spoke of The Wheel is based on a very important part of our Biography Based Care® philosophy. Persons with dementia (including Alzheimer's) are still capable of enjoying a sense of accomplishment and self-worth. Meeting your loved one's need for a sense of purpose can be accomplished by including them in daily tasks that incorporate familiar routines and skill sets that are still accessible to them. Involve them in decision-making and ask for their help whenever possible while setting them up for a successful outcome. This is about helping your loved one feel useful, helpful, that they matter and, more importantly, they are not a burden.

☐ Incorporate every day activities with age appropriate endeavors such as cooking, gardening, cleaning, sweeping, and polishing silver or shoes, hanging up the wash, sorting socks, arranging jewelry into boxes. These are routine tasks that your loved one probably participated in every day before the onset of symptoms. Create space for your loved one to continue to participate in familiar tasks built around the parts of the activity that they can still do. Many of these activities can be done successfully with your loved one if they are broken down into simple routine steps.

☐ Use the Biography tool in Chapter 2 to identify the activities that would offer the most meaningful experience for your loved one. Pick things that are sure to be accomplished easily with the least amount of frustration.

☐ Our loved one's career can be a treasure trove of ideas for activities. For many persons with dementia (including Alzheimer's), one of the last times they truly felt needed, capable and in control may have been when they were professionally active before retirement or when they were running their household. If your loved one was a secretary, ask them to help you put stamps on your letters. If they were an accountant, have them help you "pay the bills" by involving them in writing down numbers or handling a calculator.

☐ If your loved one never worked outside the home, or relates to a time when they had young children to care for, consider asking for their help in tasks that relate back to parenting. Have your loved one go with you to pick up kids or grandkids from school, making "school" lunches (even if you are the only two eating them out of those brown paper bags). Create space for interaction with children often. Some families and senior living communities have also reported positive outcomes when using life-like doll babies that your loved one can "care for."

☐ Encourage independence as much as possible. Helping your loved one brush their own teeth, get dressed or read the paper, for example, can help them feel more in control and less helpless. Give them examples by showing or telling them a couple of ways that something could be done and then let them pick what works best for them. If no harm can come from their choices, let them have a little autonomy in completing tasks. If when they set the table, there are three extra plates and no silverware, no big deal, it's an easy fix. If they are done brushing their teeth and proudly put away a dry toothbrush after drinking a glass of water in the bathroom, praise the effort and try to ask them to show you with a toothpaste-laden brush you prepare how to do it so you can learn too.

☐ Give your loved one the gift of decision making when possible. Let them pick out their clothing, meals, what music they'd like to hear, what activity they'd enjoy, etc. Protecting your loved one's ability to make choices is a great way to engage them in planning your shared days together. Make it easier for your loved one to make decisions by offering a choice of two things which can be less overwhelming than open-ended questions like "what would you like for dinner?" or "what would you like to do today?"

☐ Ask for help from your loved one often. Let them know that they are needed and that you value their advice, opinion, experience, helping hands, etc. Offer praise and recognition often so that they feel more comfortable participating. Let them know that you really need their ideas and want their input. Ask them to show or tell you how to do something. Even if what they are saying or doing doesn't make sense, go with the flow and be sure to praise them for trying to "help" you. Let your loved one know how much their contribution helps.

CHAPTER 20

Alzheimer's Adapted Activity Ideas: Social

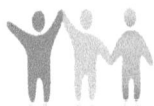

SOCIAL

The Social spoke of The Wheel is about how your loved one interacts with other people (including you). It may not mean what it used to before the onset of the disease, but there are still plenty of great ways to connect with your loved one through specific, guided interactions and activities with you, your family and friends. There are still opportunities to connect your loved one to his/her world at large.

Storytelling therapy for people with Alzheimer's taps into creativity more so than accuracy or personal history. Begin by introducing a picture or series of pictures and invite your loved one to tell a story about what they see. Just as in art therapy, communicating about an image doesn't require remembering anything, which can be an intimidating and uncomfortable aspect of the conversation. Storytelling exercises creativity, gives emotional release, and provides caregivers with interesting insights into the life and mind of the person living with dementia (including Alzheimer's).

In storytelling therapy, as in art therapy, the key is letting the person with Alzheimer's take the lead once the activity is introduced. Simply help the story along by asking basic open-ended questions.

- Use a coffee table book, magazines, greeting or post cards with large, easy to see images. At a time when your loved one feels relaxed, and things are quiet, with no distractions, look at the images together and use them as conversation starters. Ask your loved one questions about the pictures that don't sound like a quiz, with right or wrong answers. Rather solicit their opinion, asking "which of these holiday cookies looks the prettiest to you" or "where do you think this couple in the picture is going?" Let your loved one steer the conversation and talk or look at whatever captures their attention.

▫ Reminiscence therapy for persons differs from storytelling, which doesn't specifically involve memories. Reminiscence therapy invites a person with cognitive impairment to exercise their long-term memory by encouraging them to share positive recollections from younger days or familiar times. Especially in the earlier stages of the disease, your loved one may still remember and enjoy talking about their childhood or young adult years. Old photo albums, letters, memorabilia, movies, and music are great tools to help bring the "good old days" forward into the present.

▫ Focus conversations on the parts of their past that they do recall with ease. Exploring positive memories help can improve your loved one's mood, encourage verbalization, and raise self-esteem. Keep the energy relaxed and reassuring so that your loved one doesn't feel like they are being tested or quizzed. When family and friends are visiting, this is a great activity for them to participate in with your loved one. You might just learn things about your loved one that you didn't know or didn't remember. Record the new and familiar stories your loved one shares on voice or video recorder, or jot down some notes to preserve them for you and your family to treasure and reflect on in the future.

▫ Encourage family, friends and caregivers to initiate caring interactions with the person and to continue the essence of a normal relationship. Visitors should continue to greet, talk with and interact with your loved one. When conversations begin to get tougher, coach others to simply smile or reach for your loved one's hand, offer a hug or share a cup of coffee with them. Their very nearness and attempts to engage your loved one (versus talk around them as if they aren't there) will do a lot to support self-esteem and a sense of belonging.

▫ Plan and involve your loved one in activities and social situations that continue past interests and lifestyle even though the activity may need to be adapted. Set your loved one up for success by practicing the activities ahead of time before they are in a new environment or with more people around than they are used to. Be sure to offer lots of reassuring words and gestures to combat the anxiety that can be felt when your loved one could be experiencing a higher degree of uncertainty in social situations.

☐ Encourage adult day program participation so that your loved one may continue to have opportunities to remain active, involved and engaged with others. Check your local yellow pages or web listings for senior day programs that specialize in serving persons with dementia (including Alzheimer's). Many will send you a calendar of activity offerings that you can review ahead of time. Before you have your loved one attend for a trial period, be sure to talk to adult day care center staff about your loved one's specific health and social needs before you decide to give it a try. Check with your family physician or medical provider to see if this may be a good option for your loved one and be sure to disclose fully to the day center staff any special needs or concerns (such as wandering, needing assistance with toileting or medications etc.) so that they can better plan for a successful experience.

☐ Alert others in social situations discreetly that your loved one has some cognitive impairment (e.g., business sized cards from the Alzheimer's Association that advise that the person you are with has dementia (including Alzheimer's), so they can work with you to make the situation go smoothly. This can be very helpful, not just in social situations with family and friends but also when out at the grocery store, pharmacy, restaurant or even dentist and eye doctor visits.

☐ Utilize pictures, memorabilia, favorite object or activity supplies to enhance and create positive interaction during visits. Make visitors more comfortable by modeling or showing them how to engage your loved one. Most importantly set the tone that no matter what happens or what is said, you are happy to have visits for your loved one. If words don't make sense, your loved one's own child's faces seem unfamiliar or a tense moment occurs, let them know that this doesn't define or diminish the relationship that you all share. Personify a "go with the flow attitude" so your loved one and others can take their cues from you. Ensure that the overall takeaway from these social interactions is that you and your loved one got to be with people that care about your loved one. What did or didn't happen doesn't matter as much as the fact that you got to be with one another.

☐   Help family and friends realize not to take your loved one's actions or comments personally when behavior symptoms occur - teach them strategies for moving past awkward moments and maintaining a sense of humor. Let them know that sometimes it is the disease process and not your loved one behaving in this manner and encourage them to reflect on their relationship with your loved one over the span of its entirety—all of the weeks, months or years that they've had together not just the present version of their bond.

CHAPTER 21

Alzheimer's Adapted Activity Ideas: Encouraging Intellectual Engagement

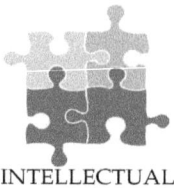

INTELLECTUAL

The Intellectual Engagement spoke of The Wheel focuses on creating positive ways to work within your loved one's abilities to stimulate memory and thinking. This is a fun and playful way to connect while gently encouraging your loved one to participate in a wide range of activities. There are lots of choices here, from reminiscing and trivia to simple sorting and easy memory games depending on what stage of the disease process your loved one is in. The success here lies solely in your loved one's participation. It's all about the "doing" and not the "completing".

☐ Physical games that encourage hand-eye coordination can meet both physical and intellectual needs. Look for games that require a low level of fitness but offer a chance of meeting a goal. Bean bags tossed into a pail, croquet, indoor foam or plastic versions of darts, bowling or horseshoes are also great choices.

☐ Current affairs are a good place to have conversations that combine what's happening today with memories from yesteryear. For example, use upcoming elections to reminisce about favorite presidents. Use current reports about NASA and the space program to engage in discussion about the first moon landing.

☐ Faces and places are a fun way to take a virtual tour through your loved one's life story. With photo albums, magazines and postcards, talk about previous homes, vacations or school friends. Gather older photos that represent a time that is more familiar to your loved one. For example, they may not recognize the 45-year-old woman caring for them as their daughter, but a picture of that same woman as a little girl on her first day of school may elicit some pleasant memories. This can also be played with flashcards/pictures of animals and objects that your loved one can then identify or name.

☐ Word games can be a very enjoyable way to foster a sense of success while having a lot of fun. Think of familiar phrases, songs, movies or books and begin but don't finish the names or phrases. For example, ask your loved one to finish the song lyric: "Take me out to the _____"or for a movie title such as "Gone with the _____"or a famous actor "Humphrey _____" and the like. The more you can use a particular area of interest for your loved one, the more likely they'll be to participate in this game. Try the alphabet song by getting it started and letting your loved one join in "A, B, C, D, E, F, G, _____". These games can be played by writing things out on a piece of paper or just saying them aloud depending on which your loved one likes best.

☐ Being creative is also another wonderful example of engaging the intellect and a way that we often overlook. The process that is drawing, painting, writing, making collages, doing craft projects or decorating cookies all engage your loved one in thinking about colors, shapes, textures, tastes, themes or feelings.

☐ Categorizing or sorting objects is an activity that can be easily adapted for most stages in the disease process. Take care to ensure adequate supervision when sorting smaller items that can be ingested. Socks, buttons, nut/bolts, silverware, poker chips, playing cards and the like can all be sorted in a variety of ways. With playing cards, for instance, a higher functioning person may be able to put suits in numeric order while later in the disease process, the goal may simply be to sort black and red cards into piles.

☐ Orientation is about interacting around the time, place and person. This type of activity is best suited for those that are comfortable with a question like "What season is it when we see red, yellow and orange leaves outside?" Or "what is your full name" or "where were you born"? Have some flexibility around modifying questions to help your loved one succeed. If possible stay away from questions that begin with words such as, "How" or "Why" as they can be perceived as aggressive and may potentially create some frustration or defensiveness if your loved one is unable to easily explain themselves.

☐ Using money is an activity that can be done without actually purchasing anything or going outside the home. Your loved one can help you sort money by denomination (coins are perfect for this as they are different shapes and color such as pennies versus nickels) or practice making change or gathering the amount needed to "buy" something from your pantry. Monopoly or toy money can be also used instead of the real thing.

☐ Number games let your loved one put numbers in order by playing what comes next. Like word games, you can play these by writing on a piece of paper or saying them aloud. For example, start by saying the sequence "2, 4, 6, 8" and then listen to what comes next. Try writing 1, 2, 3, and 4 on a piece of paper and let your loved one finish. Sort playing cards into odd and even numbers or put them in numeric order. Simple addition, subtraction or saying the multiplication tables are good ways to engage higher functioning loved ones in earlier stages. For those further along in the disease process, you may like to count crackers at lunchtime as you serve them or make piles of grapes, nuts or other edibles as you snack and play.

☐ Trivia is another one of those highly personal activities that really are more fun when they are specific to your loved one. Asking a sports fan Oscar-winning best picture trivia may cause more frustration than pleasure for example. Knowing your loved ones' areas of interest can help ensure that they are challenged but not upset by the questions you are solving together. Give lots of hints and praise and jump in if they get stuck. There are a number of board games and senior editions of trivia cards, but you can also make up your own for free with a little imagination. Keep the questions as simple as you can, and again, stick with topics that your loved one talks about or remembers well. Such as: "Name a baseball team in New York" or "What color was the _____ Rose of Texas?"

☐ As with any of the activity ideas previously shared, feel free to play intellectual games with your loved one as long as they are having fun and pay attention to verbal feedback and body language to avoid building frustration.

SECTION TWO:
Coping Strategies for Care Partners

CHAPTER 22

Making Time for Moments That Matter

As a care partner, so much of your day is necessarily about the tasks, the "to-do" list. It's normal and completely understandable that those day-to-day, "have to do" tasks have become the day's primary focus.

Some family care partners wake up each morning with a prioritized plan of how they'd like the day to go. The execution of duties like ensuring that medications are taken, showers or baths are given safely, toileting accomplished, laundry, meals, dishes and appointments are taken care of and that adequate supervision is provided at all times for their loved one often 24 hours per day, become the daily priorities. The new normal may feel a lot like just getting through the day.

That "to-do" list (either recorded on paper, computer or kept mentally) is never far from most care partner's thoughts. Some review it in their minds as the last thing they think about before retiring each night. Weighing what was accomplished and what wasn't. Reflecting on what they did do, didn't do, what did get done, could've gotten done or should've been done in a kind of self-imposed audit enacted by internal order to measure and gauge their level of success or capability as a care partner when often the only witness to their efforts is no longer able to recognize or appreciate all that they do.

The daily dance with how much you did or didn't get done and how you feel about yourself can be an emotionally draining aspect of caregiving. This chapter is about challenging the definition of successful caregiving to include not just what you do for your loved one, but how you do it.

Consider The Wheel again for a moment. Meeting your loved one's physical needs (bathing, dressing, grooming, medications, meals etc. represented by the Physical spoke of The Wheel), are just 1/6 of our loved one's whole person needs. Yet, supporting these physical needs likely account for the majority of most care partners' day leaving little time to meet other equally important elements. Some family care partners may feel like they spend up to 90% of their caregiving time devoted to their loved one's physical health and safety. Others report that it already feels like there aren't enough hours in the day or that the idea of "adding" anything else is too overwhelming.

While meeting your loved one's health and safety needs are of utmost importance, there are other aspects (Spiritual/Calm, Emotional, Sense of Purpose, Social, and Intellectual Engagement) of their care as well, that, when met, can have a very positive impact on their quality of life and yours.

If you are like most care partners I've spoken to over the years, you agree with the idea of spending more quality time together, but have trouble finding the time and energy to do so. On the following pages are some quick tips to help you carve out more space in an already overcrowded day to make time for moments that matter.

- ☐ Use a calendar to organize the day. A customizable Dementia (including Alzheimer's) Weekly Care Plan can be found in Chapter 23 to help you plan out your day and budget your time according to your priorities and needs. With dementia (including Alzheimer's), the only thing we can plan on is that most times nothing will go exactly as planned. However, having a plan does help. It can better help you get back on track and minimize the disruptions to your routine when they occur (and disruptions will occur).

- ☐ Put laughing ahead of laundry (at least sometimes!). Part of your daily goals should include at least one activity or interaction designed just for fun. Your loved one has likely lost the ability to self-initiate the satisfaction of their own needs, including the pursuit of pleasure or fun. Make it a point to plan on setting time aside for this type of experience, whatever that may be. Studies have shown that if we write our goals down, they are more likely to be achieved. Try making a fun interaction as much of a daily priority as medications, toileting, and meals. Try it for just one week and see how it goes. Making it important to you increases the chances that it will happen for your loved one. Bottom line, if you don't make it a priority, it probably won't happen.

☐ Put the past in the past. Hands down, one of the saddest things I've heard from families about the reasons their loved one "just sits there" or "doesn't do anything anymore" surprisingly wasn't related to the disease process. When I dug a little deeper, I learned it was often because their well-meaning but overworked care partners just stopped trying to engage them in activities for a variety of understandable reasons. Try to look objectively at any barriers on your end that may be preventing you from facilitating fun activities and interactions. There are a lot of potential barriers to having the strength and energy to put on your "pom-poms" yet again to cheering yourselves on and up by dreaming up new and different activities to keep you both connected and entertained. Maybe your loved one lacked interest last time you tried to engage them in an activity, maybe you were just too exhausted, maybe your feelings were still hurt because of the way you were spoken to or treated yesterday. Perhaps they may not have appreciated all that you tried to do in inviting them to participate in something you really thought they might enjoy, only to be rebuffed. Maybe at that moment, whatever you were trying just didn't work. This is where you wipe the slate clean and remember that what happened yesterday was yesterday. Your loved one may not even remember what was said. They are probably completely unaware that you are harboring some hurt on account of their behavior. Don't get discouraged. Not everybody feels like doing something all the time, it doesn't mean that your loved one might not want or is unable to engage with you any longer. Today is a new day. A whole new chance to begin again, a fresh start. Don't let past practices prevent you from future successes. Keep trying! Attempt different activity ideas, alternate times of day, and change approaches. It's okay to keep starting over.

☐ Attitude is everything. Look for ways to make the mundane magical. Have a plan for when you feel that you are starting to get stressed out and feeling overwhelmed. "Stop" and do something fun for a few minutes. Think about all the people you have met over your lifetime. Do you remember special family, friends, schoolmates, neighbors, teachers, and others you've met over a lifetime? Chances are the ones that stand out, your favorites, are remembered that way not because of what they did for you, but because of how they made you feel. We remember the kind of person who makes going to the grocery store a grand adventure because when you're with them everything seems more fun. We cherish this kind of person. Who never makes you feel like you're a bother, the person who looks forward to seeing you every time you meet and the person who loves you unconditionally and thinks that you can do no wrong. Who wouldn't want to know and spend their day with a person like that? Do you know a person like that? Are you a person like that? It's okay to be a bit whimsical, a little silly and a whole lot ridiculous sometimes. Look for fun wherever you can find it and try to find the humor in all things. Be the person you would want to spend your day with and your loved one will have a better experience with you and you with them.

☐ Get a jump start by doing tomorrow's tasks tonight. At the end of a long day, the last thing on your mind is probably trying to fit in "just one more thing". Throwing a load of laundry in the washer, loading the dinner dishes and running the dishwasher or even setting the table for breakfast may be worth the extra effort tonight to give you a little extra time tomorrow.

☐ Look for ways to save time on chores. Try paper plates to decrease dishwashing, prepare crock pot meals and make more than you need and then portion out and freeze them into individual meals that can be thawed when needed. When making something (salads, sandwiches, soups, snacks) always try to make extra if it will keep. If you're going to go to all the trouble of making it, why not make enough for you both to have enjoyed a few meals from your efforts instead of just one? When doing laundry, put clothing away in sets or complete outfits. On one hanger have a shirt, pants undergarments and socks draped over the shoulder so dressing can be a grab and go task that doesn't require thinking about what matches or fits or is clean because these items have already been selected and grouped together. It also cuts down on time we spend looking for certain pieces of clothing.

☐ Start small. Have reasonable expectations. Instead of trying to meet one need from each spoke each day at first, try picking one per day. Always try to set aside 10-15 minutes per day for an enjoyable activity. As you find what works best for you and your loved one, you can gradually start adding additional times for activities. Remember, this is for fun…not an obligatory "to do" list but rather a "let's see how many ways we can find to play today" list!

☐ Find common interests. Use the Biography Based Care® Biography form in Chapter 2 to reflect on your loved one's past careers, hobbies, interests and favorite activities. When possible look for overlap with the pursuits that you enjoy as well. You'll both get much more out of your shared experiences if they are something that you can both appreciate.

☐ Have everything you need on hand. Preparation is key. A lot of our activity ideas found in the appendix are purposely built around using things you'll likely already have around the house and have accumulated over the years. Our activities are meant to get the most mileage out of the least materials, the most interaction with the least amount of stuff. We believe meaningful moments happen in the interaction, not because of the inanimate objects. Having said that, you will want some activity supplies readily available. It's a good idea to think about what you want those to be so you can gather or purchase them ahead of time. Make sure that not having activity items readily available isn't a barrier when you and your loved one are both in the right mindset to participate in a shared experience.

☐ Involve others. Play dates aren't just for kids! Meeting another family care partners in the right environment for a chance to visit and participate in an activity alongside another caregiver and tier loved one is a great way to share ideas and promote socializing for both of you. This can be done through classes at Alzheimer's specific Adult Day Care Centers, Alzheimer's Association, church support groups or networking on your own. Check online or in your local yellow pages or community services directory for offerings in your area that may help you and your loved one enjoy all of the benefits of participating in the fun without the hassle of planning.

☐ Set aside a block of alone time each day. Make time for you, whether it is having quiet time with a cup of coffee and a good book in the mornings before your loved one wakes up or browsing the Internet while they nap, be sure to set aside time each day to do something enjoyable for yourself. Part of making time for moments that matter is also giving yourself permission to take time for you. Even if it's just a few minutes to take a bath, light your favorite candle, use the good moisturizing lotion (you know, the one you've been saving), listening to your favorite music from high school or opening that great bottle of wine. It's okay. Take the time to make a moment that matters just for you! You deserve it!

CHAPTER 23

Getting the Help that You Want on Your Terms

The impact of being a primary care partner for a person with dementia (including Alzheimer's) can have a negative impact on your emotional and physical well-being. Often care partners report feeling exhausted, but note that asking for help feels like a failure and receiving help feels like they're a burden. It's not always the best solution to single-handedly sustain meeting your loved one's needs (as well as your own) 24-hours per day indefinitely. Consider these solutions to make yourself and others feel more comfortable when you alone are not enough to accomplish all of the necessary tasks on your "to do" list.

☐ Divide up your "to-do" list. There are some things that you or your loved one may not feel comfortable having others help with (bathing, dressing, medications or even personal laundry). It's okay to be specific about the areas where help would be most welcome. Dividing your "to do" list into those areas that you really need to be in charge of and those areas that the helping hands of others (picking up a medication, running out to get milk, etc.) would be really appreciated, this may help you be more prepared and confident in answering the question, the next time someone asks "what can I do to help?" See our "What Would Would Really Help Me" flyer on page 150 or download your own copy to share with family and friends on our website's homepage: www. whencaringtakescourage.com.

☐ Create space for others to participate in care. Sometimes it's a good idea to let others help because you may need a little break or because you have so much to do that it's going to take more than one person to physically get through all of the tasks that need completing. At other times, it's a good idea to let others help because it meets their need to feel useful, to feel connected to you, and/or to your loved one.

☐ Have a plan to get extra help BEFORE you need it. Emergencies can and do happen often and unexpectedly. Plan ahead by identifying who can be counted on to help in a pinch. Ask family or close friends if they would be available in the event of an emergency.

☐ Endeavor to create partner relationships with family and a few close friends that you can trust and call upon when needed. It can be an invaluable help to have a prepared back–up plan. You never know when you'll be in a situation where you'll need a ride, when you need someone to help with an errand or help stay with your loved one. Even if you don't want to give yourself permission for a break now and then, an emergency or illness may make asking for help a necessity.

☐ Meet with and "train" helpers before you need them! Meet with the person(s) you've identified ahead of time to go over any questions that they may have and share needed caregiver "how to's" specific to your loved one.

☐ Schedule regular or routine tasks. Be strategic in your planning by grouping errands based on geographical area, tasks that can be planned to occur around MD and other appointments and map out a plan of the day or week if that helps. Laundry may need to be done several times per week, but planning out when the best TIME is to do it (i.e. when your loved one is sleeping or when they are most likely to have the energy and inclination to enjoy helping you fold fresh warm towels). They can help you identify days of the week and times of day that work best for you based on the rhythm of life and activity in your home for you and your loved one.

☐ Know the difference between WANT to do and HAVE to do. Reflect objectively on what really NEEDS to get done and what tasks are just things that you WANT to get done. Caregiving for a person with cognitive impairment means that things are constantly changing around you and the more flexible you are the less stressed you'll become. Get comfortable with changing plans and priorities as often as needed. It's okay to let the little things go in favor of focusing on overall priorities for care such as safety and wellbeing.

☐ Team up with other care partners. Consider working with primary caregivers to share tasks and errands like shopping, pharmacy and medical appointments when possible.

☐ Check out both volunteer and paid organizations in your area. Your physician, The Alzheimer's Association, Area Agency on Aging, Adult Day Care, Home Care, Assisted Living, Companion Care, or Senior Center are some of the organizations that you may want to explore.

☐ Focus on the greater good. Don't let feelings, such as guilt, need to be in control, or hesitancy to be perceived as a bother prevent you from seeking the support you and your loved one need to have the best possible day. Successful caregiving means effectively and safely meeting needs on a 24 hour basis which is difficult for any one person to sustain for long periods of time.

☐ Have a plan. There are a lot of studies currently that emphasize the benefit of creating routines for people with dementia (including Alzheimer's). Having a loosely based game plan around time frames for meals, bath/shower times, medications and household chores and errands can help you plot out your time, create a familiar pattern for your loved one and make it easier for another person to help out because they'll know what's "going on." Having said that, there are going to be times when the plan doesn't happen as scheduled because you or your loved one may feel like doing something else, and that's okay. This is more about having a framework of things that you'd like to have happen, the when and how of these things is up to you to accomplish them in the way that makes the best sense given the situation.

On the following pages (pages 140 and 141) you'll find Biography Based Care's two page Dementia (Including Alzheimer's) Care Weekly Care Planner to give you some ideas of what things you may want to plan for daily and weekly. Don't feel pressured to provide every caregiving task listed, this is a compilation of best practices for your review.

Care partners have used the Weekly Care Planner a few different ways, such as:

- ☐ Determining where they are currently spending most of their time/day by placing an "x" in the box at the end of each day to correspond with what actually occurred.

- ☐ Deciding how they want to spend their day by placing an "X" in the box that corresponds to what they want to do.

- ☐ Creating opportunities for family and friends to participate in helping the primary care partner meet their loved one's care by engaging them in setting/reviewing care goals each week.

- ☐ Communicating with home health staff and care aides what care you'd like your loved one to receive, or showing your loved one's primary care and other medical providers a better picture of current care needs.

Caregiving tasks on the Weekly Care Planner have been divided into the categories below to make it easier to identify and find the tasks most relevant to you:

- ☐ Medications
- ☐ Toileting
- ☐ Bathing/grooming
- ☐ Meals
- ☐ Life Enrichment
- ☐ Household Chores

Taking a moment to review the sample weekly care planner can help you ask yourself the tough questions that will help you adjust your plan as you see fit. Here are some things to consider:

- ✓ Are your loved one's needs bring met?
- ✓ Are they safe?
- ✓ Are you physically and emotionally able to carry out all of the care tasks required on your own?
- ✓ What parts of your day together are most fulfilling for you both?
- ✓ Are there parts of the day/tasks that others could help with so that you have more quality time with your loved one?
- ✓ Are there any gaps in care needed and care available?
- ✓ Would you and your loved one benefit from some help (paid or unpaid) from others?
- ✓ Do you have enough time left in the day to take care of yourself?

Biography ♥ Based Care
Dementia (including Alzheimer's) Weekly Care Plan

Medications Toileting Bathing/grooming Meals Life Enrichment Household Chores

Care tasks include:	Sunday	Monday	Tuesday	Wednesday	Thursday	Friday	Saturday
AM Toileting or Continence Care							
AM Dressing							
AM Grooming							
Bath or Shower							
AM Medications							
Breakfast Meal Prep							
Breakfast Meal							
Breakfast Dishes							
AM Life Enrichment Activity							
Make AM Snack Together							
AM Snack and Hydration							
Midday Toileting or Continence Care							
Midday Medications							
Lunch Meal Prep							
Lunch Meal							
Lunch Dishes							
Midday Life Enrichment Activity							
Afternoon Toileting or Continence Care							

Biography ❤ Based Care

Dementia (including Alzheimer's) Weekly Care Plan

Identify which of these care tasks apply to your loved one. Use this worksheet to help plan your week and determine where you might want/need additional assistance.

Categories: Medications | Toileting | Bathing/grooming | Meals | Life Enrichment | Household Chores

Care tasks include:	Sunday	Monday	Tuesday	Wednesday	Thursday	Friday	Saturday
Make Afternoon Snack Together							
Afternoon Snack and Hydration							
Calming and Comfort Time							
Dinner Meal Prep							
Evening Toileting or Continence Care							
Dinner Meal							
Dinner Dishes							
Dinner Medications							
Evening Life Enrichment Activity							
Make Bedtime Snack Together							
Bedtime Snack							
Bedtime Grooming							
Bedtime Medications							
Bedtime Dressing/Undressing							
Bedtime Toileting or Continence Care							
Laundry Day(s)							
Grocery Shopping Day(s)							
Housecleaning Day(s)							
Pharmacy Trip							
MD/Medical appointments							

Another way to take a closer look at the amount of care your loved one needs is with the Care Needs Calculators. They are designed to be utilized as a general guide and make no assurances or guarantees regarding your loved one's safety. Each family's experience with Alzheimer's/Dementia is different. Not only is the journey of those living with the disease specific to them, but also each caregiver's experience is as unique as their skill set, physical ability and energy level. You are ultimately responsible for the safety of your loved one and as such should consult with your loved one's physician and care providers when making determinations regarding the best setting and staffing to meet individual and specific care needs. The Care Needs Calculator(s) are intended to give general information to help support you and your health care team in identifying care needs and the amount of time and support your loved one may require.

It is recommended that you bring your completed Care Needs Calculator to your medical appointments and review the results with your medical providers. This tool can also be used as a starting point for family discussions about how best to meet your loved one's needs. It is a "best practice" to update the Care Needs Calculator at least once per quarter, or any time significant changes occur so that adjustments in care can be made to accommodate your loved one's changing needs throughout the course of the disease process.

 The first step is to determine how much time you spend helping your loved one with specific tasks. Secondly, what kind of help are you providing to support them in successfully completing their activities of daily living (cueing or total assistance for example). Biography Based Care's Care Needs Calculators are designed to help you objectively determine these two things.

You only need to complete one version of the care needs calculator.

The Abbreviated Care Needs Calculator (page 143) is a shorter version for those that have a good idea already how and where they are spending their time caregiving.

The Comprehensive Care Needs Calculator (pages 144-149) walks readers through their caregiving duties in more detail to better help caregivers how and where they spend their time caring for their loved one.

Abbreviated Care Needs Calculator

CARE TASKS	Total Hours PER WEEK
BATHING Cueing, reminders, physical assistance or hands on help with personal safety, fall risk prevention, skin/injury check, washing hair/body and overall supervision	
DRESSING Cueing, reminders, physical assistance or hands on help for: dressing and undressing, personal laundry	
GROOMING (Cueing, reminders, physical assistance or hands on help to clean/wash: hair, teeth, nails, ears, face, feet, shave etc. Getting them to wear glasses, hearing aids. Obtaining weight regularly)	
MEALS (Meal prep, shopping, cooking, cleaning, reminders, cueing for eating, safety and supervision related to diet and swallowing)	
MEDICATIONS AND APPOINTMENTS Medication supervision, cueing, reminders, re-ordering. Coordination of calls with MD's and pharmacies and insurance providers, travel to/from	
TOILETING Reminders, cueing, or physical assistance to use the toilet or commode. Use of incontinence products, additional laundry, personal grooming/clean up	
HOUSEHOLD MANAGEMENT Laundering of linens, groceries and shopping, banking, bill paying, medical appointment coordination, yard work, transportation, home/auto upkeep	
SAFETY Decreasing fall risks, wander guard, reminders to use assistive devices i.e. cane, walker, hearing aid or glasses, supervision around water, heat, cold, poison prevention	
LIFE ENRICHMENT Reminiscing, hands on leisure and recreational activities inside and outside the home, visitors, exercise, worship, socializing at home in the community	
GRAND TOTAL CAREGIVING HOURS PER WEEK (Add all areas from each row to obtain grand total of weekly caregiving hours)	
0 to 42 hours of caregiving per week	Needs may be met by single caregiver provided that the caregiver is able/willing and if no safety risk is present requiring 24 hour supervision. Dementia specific caregiver training is recommended.
43-69 hours of caregiving per week	Needs may be met by 2 caregivers provided that the caregivers are able/willing and if no safety risk is present requiring 24 hour supervision. Dementia specific caregiver training is recommended.
70-98 hours of caregiving per week	Needs may be met by 3 caregivers provided that the caregivers are able/willing and if no safety risk is present requiring 24 hour supervision. Dementia specific caregiver training is recommended.
99+ hours of caregiving tasks per week on average	**24-hour supervision by an awake, specially trained, dementia care provider is required.**
SAFETY RISK/DANGER TO SELF OR OTHERS	**24-hour supervision by an awake, specially trained, dementia care provider is required.**

© 2016 Mara Botonis, excerpt from the book *"When Caring Takes Courage"*

Biography ❧ Based Care.
Comprehensive Care Needs Calculator

BATHING Choose the answer that best reflects the care that your loved one needs on average with each task. Enter a point value in only one column for each task.	Only a gentle reminder needed. Then loved one can execute the task independently 1 Point	Verbal cueing during some or all of the steps it takes for loved one to complete task 3 Points	Hands on assistance with 30% of the task needed from caregiver to complete task 5 Points	Hands on assistance with 50% of the task needed from caregiver to complete task 7 Points	Loved one is unable to complete this task and is completely dependent on caregiver 10 Points
Knowing when to bathe					
Turning on/off water safely					
Using safe water temperature					
Using soap and shampoo safely, washing hair					
Washing body/genitals					
Decreasing fall risks					
Total points each column					
Total Points this section from ALL columns	_____ Points	Multiply total points x 10 minutes= Total caregiving time per week: Bathing			

DRESSING Choose the answer that best reflects the care that your loved one needs on average with each task. Enter a point value in only one column for each task.	Only a gentle reminder needed. Then loved one can execute the task independently 1 Point	Verbal cueing during some or all of the steps it takes for loved one to complete task 3 Points	Hands on assistance with 30% of the task needed from caregiver to complete task 5 Points	Hands on assistance with 50% of the task needed from caregiver to complete task 7 Points	Loved one is unable to complete this task and is completely dependent on caregiver 10 Points
Locating clean clothes					
Assembling an entire outfit					
Identifying appropriate attire based upon activity and season/temperature					
Buttoning/zipping					
Upper body dressing					
Lower body dressing					
Donning shoes and socks					
Changing into clean clothes					
Putting clothes in hamper					
Total points each column					
Total Points this section from ALL columns	_____ Points	Multiply total points x 10 minutes= Total caregiving time per week: Dressing			

GROOMING Choose the answer that best reflects the care that your loved one needs on average with each task. Enter a point value in only one column for each task.	Only a gentle reminder needed. Then loved one can execute the task independently 1 Point	Verbal cueing during some or all of the steps it takes for loved one to complete task 3 Points	Hands on assistance with 30% of the task needed from caregiver to complete task 5 Points	Hands on assistance with 50% of the task needed from caregiver to complete task 7 Points	Loved one is unable to complete this task and is completely dependent on caregiver 10 Points
Brushing and flossing					
Brushing hair/washing face					
Clipping nails					
Shaving					
Applying make-up					
Personal hygiene					
Using hearing aid(s) or glasses if applicable					
Denture care if applicable					
Total points each column					
Total Points this section from ALL columns	_____ Points	Multiply total points x 10 minutes= Total caregiving time per week: Grooming			

MEALS Choose the answer that best reflects the care that your loved one needs on average with each task. Enter a point value in only one column for each task.	Only a gentle reminder needed. Then loved one can execute the task independently 1 Point	Verbal cueing during some or all of the steps it takes for loved one to complete task 2 Points	Hands on assistance with 30% of the task needed from caregiver to complete task 3 Points	Hands on assistance with 50% of the task needed from caregiver to complete task 4 Points	Loved one is unable to complete this task and is completely dependent on caregiver 10 Points
Recognizing hunger or thirst					
Planning a meal					
Using stove/oven safely					
Using microwave safely					
Obtaining adequate nutrition					
Using silverware/eating					
Obtaining adequate hydration					
Swallowing/chewing safely					
Proper food storage /managing expiration dates					
Cleanliness/food safety					
Total points each column					
Total Points this section from ALL columns	_____ Points	Multiply total points x 10 minutes= Total caregiving time per week: Meals			

MEDICATIONS Choose the answer that best reflects the care that your loved one needs on average with each task. Enter a point value in only one column for each task.	Only a gentle reminder needed. Then loved one can execute the task independently 1 Point	Verbal cueing during some or all of the steps it takes for loved one to complete task 3 Points	Hands on assistance with 30% of the task needed from caregiver to complete task 5 Points	Hands on assistance with 50% of the task needed from caregiver to complete task 7 Points	Loved one is unable to complete this task and is completely dependent on caregiver 10 Points
Taking medications as prescribed/on time					
Identifying different medications/why each medication is being taken					
Articulating adverse medication reactions					
Swallowing medication safely					
Asking for non-routine medications due to pain or discomfort					
Communicating with pharmacy/MD as needed regarding medications					
Total points each column					
Total Points this section from ALL columns	_____ Points	Multiply total points x 10 minutes= Total caregiving time per week: Medications			

TOILETING Choose the answer that best reflects the care that your loved one needs on average with each task. Enter a point value in only one column for each task.	Only a gentle reminder needed. Then loved one can execute the task independently 1 Point	Verbal cueing during some or all of the steps it takes for loved one to complete task 3 Points	Hands on assistance with 30% of the task needed from caregiver to complete task 5 Points	Hands on assistance with 50% of the task needed from caregiver to complete task 7 Points	Loved one is unable to complete this task and is completely dependent on caregiver 10 Points
Identifying urge to toilet					
Using toilet for voiding					
Proper hygiene after toileting					
Identifying/resolving soiled clothing when needed					
Changing incontinence pads if applicable					
Articulating any pain or discomfort with toileting					
Proper hand washing					
Total points each column					
Total Points this section from ALL columns	_____ Points	Multiply total points x 10 minutes= Total caregiving time per week: Toileting			

HOUSEHOLD MANAGEMENT Choose the answer that best reflects the care that your loved one needs on average with each task. Enter a point value in only one column for each task.	Only a gentle reminder needed. Then loved one can execute the task independently 1 Point	Verbal cueing during some or all of the steps it takes for loved one to complete task 3 Points	Hands on assistance with 30% of the task needed from caregiver to complete task 5 Points	Hands on assistance with 50% of the task needed from caregiver to complete task 7 Points	Loved one is unable to complete this task and is completely dependent on caregiver 10 Points
Laundry/housecleaning					
Grocery shopping					
Driving safely/car care					
Banking/money management					
Managing mail and bills					
Pet care (if applicable)					
Home repairs/yard work					
Neighborhood navigation, traveling safely to/from home					
Managing appointments					
Total points each column					
Total Points this section from ALL columns	_____ Points	Multiply total points x 10 minutes= Total caregiving time per week: Household Mgmt.			

LIFE ENRICHMENT Choose the answer that best reflects the care that your loved one needs on average with each task. Enter a point value in only one column for each task.	Only a gentle reminder needed. Then loved one can execute the task independently 1 Point	Verbal cueing during some or all of the steps it takes for loved one to complete task 3 Points	Hands on assistance with 30% of the task needed from caregiver to complete task 5 Points	Hands on assistance with 50% of the task needed from caregiver to complete task 7 Points	Loved one is unable to complete this task and is completely dependent on caregiver 10 Points
Ability to self-initiate pleasurable activities					
Engages in 3-5 pleasurable activities per day					
Daily physical exercise as able					
Daily social activity					
Daily recreational activity					
Daily purposeful project					
Daily spiritual or calming/comfort time					
Total points each column					
Total Points this section from ALL columns	_____ Points	Multiply total points x 10 minutes= Total caregiving time per week: Life Enrichment			

Biography ♥ Based Care®

Comprehensive Care Needs Calculator Totals

	Minutes		Hour(s)
Total minutes **BATHING** section	_____ Minutes	Divide total minutes this section by 60= Total caregiving hours this section	____:____ Hour(s)
Total minutes **DRESSING** section	_____ Minutes	Divide total minutes this section by 60= Total caregiving hours this section	____:____ Hour(s)
Total minutes **GROOMING** section	_____ Minutes	Divide total minutes this section by 60= Total caregiving hours this section	____:____ Hour(s)
Total minutes **MEALS** section	_____ Minutes	Divide total minutes this section by 60= Total caregiving hours this section	____:____ Hour(s)
Total minutes **MEDICATIONS** section	_____ Minutes	Divide total minutes this section by 60= Total caregiving hours this section	____:____ Hour(s)
Total minutes **TOILETING** section	_____ Minutes	Divide total minutes this section by 60= Total caregiving hours this section	____:____ Hour(s)
Total minutes **HOUSEHOLD MANAGEMENT** section	_____ Minutes	Divide total minutes this section by 60= Total caregiving hours this section	____:____ Hour(s)
Total minutes **LIFE ENRICHMENT** section	_____ Minutes	Divide total minutes this section by 60= Total caregiving hours this section	____:____ Hour(s)
GRAND TOTAL ALL MINUTES from ALL columns	_____ **TOTAL MINUTES**	**GRAND TOTAL** Divide Total Minutes by 60= Total Hours spent Caregiving Per Week	____:____ **TOTAL CAREGIVING HOURS ON AVERAGE PER WEEK**

SAFETY Circle the answer that best reflects the care that your loved one needs on average with each task. If your loved one needs even minimal assistance with any of the items below, 24 hours supervision is recommend to decrease the risk of injury/harm.	Gentle reminder needed. Then loved one can execute the task independently	Verbal cueing during some or all of the steps it takes for loved one to complete task	Hands on assistance with 30% of the task needed from caregiver to complete task	Hands on assistance with 50% of the task needed from caregiver to complete task	Loved one is unable to complete this task and is completely dependent on caregiver
Decreasing fall risk, safely navigating around trip hazards and using stairs	*24 hour Supervision is Needed	*24 hour Supervision is Needed	*24 hour Supervision is Needed	*24 hour Supervision is Needed	*24 hour Supervision is Needed
Using cane/walker or wheelchair consistently	*24 hour Supervision is Needed	*24 hour Supervision is Needed	*24 hour Supervision is Needed	*24 hour Supervision is Needed	*24 hour Supervision is Needed
Wandering or eloping outside of home or into unsafe areas	*24 hour Supervision is Needed	*24 hour Supervision is Needed	*24 hour Supervision is Needed	*24 hour Supervision is Needed	*24 hour Supervision is Needed
Ability to avoid situations that may result in physical harm to self or others	*24 hour Supervision is Needed	*24 hour Supervision is Needed	*24 hour Supervision is Needed	*24 hour Supervision is Needed	*24 hour Supervision is Needed
Seeking emergency or routine assistance appropriately when warranted	*24 hour Supervision is Needed	*24 hour Supervision is Needed	*24 hour Supervision is Needed	*24 hour Supervision is Needed	*24 hour Supervision is Needed

Biography ❧ Based Care®
Comprehensive Care Needs Calculator Summary Page

Total caregiving hours per week on average	**Up to 42 care hours per week** (average of 6 hours per day, 7 days per week)	Needs may be met by single caregiver provided that the caregiver is able/willing and if no safety risk is present requiring 24 hour supervision. Dementia specific caregiver training is recommended.
Total caregiving hours per week on average	**43 to 69 care hours per week**	Needs may be met by 2 caregivers provided that the caregivers are able/willing and if no safety risk is present requiring 24 hour supervision. Dementia specific caregiver training is recommended.
Total caregiving hours per week on average	**70 to 98 care hours per week**	Needs may be met by 3 caregivers provided that the caregivers are able/willing and if no safety risk is present requiring 24 hour supervision. Dementia specific caregiver training is recommended.
Total caregiving hours per week on average	**99 or more care hours per week**	**24 hour supervision by an awake, specially trained, dementia care provider is required.**
SAFETY RISK	**Circling any answer on the SAFETY**	**24 hour supervision by an awake, specially trained, dementia care provider is required.**

WHAT WOULD *REALLY* HELP ME...

TOP 10 Ways Family & Friends Can Help

1   **Don't feel like you need to cheer me up.** Don't feel like you have to "fix" it. There is no way to reverse Alzheimer's disease at this time. Let's just try to love each other through it.

2   **A small gesture goes a long, long way.** The gifts that matter most are the ones that help me save time and energy or are a treat that I can enjoy at home without arranging care. I don't always have time to read a book or watch a movie, or take advantage of invites to restaurant meals or spa treatments. Thank you for thinking of me, but the things that I can enjoy most often are ones that don't require me leaving home or arranging back up care. A pre-made meal or favorite dessert/snack, a mini photo album of pictures of us over the years, a soft cuddly blanket, great music, fresh flowers or a selection of teas and coffees would be so welcome.

3   **Please don't make me feel guilty.** I'm sorry I may be missing family gatherings, or not connecting with you as often as I used to. Please try to understand my whole world is turned upside down right now.

4   **Write me a note or an email.** I can't always talk on the phone or devote the time I'd like to an in-person visit. The times during the day when I'm "free" to socialize are usually only the hours when my loved one is sleeping and even then, I keep watchful eyes and listening ears tuned into what's going on around me. If you write to me, I can read it when I have time to truly enjoy it.

5   **Be patient with me when we do connect.** It may seem like I'm tired, cranky, consumed by everything Alzheimer's and dementia related and almost incapable of summoning the social graces to make "small talk". Just know that I care about you, I miss you, and I'm very interested in your life. I'm just really wiped out right now. As hard as this is for me, I wouldn't change it. Love is about being there for the other person, especially when they need you most.

6   **Reminisce with me.** I willingly, loving and without hesitation put another person first for most parts of my every day. Sometimes I feel like big parts of me get "lost", please remind me of a time before Alzheimer's and dementia entered our lives. You may be the only one in my life that I get to do this with.

7   **If you think I'm doing a good job, please tell me.** Most days I feel like I'm failing, trying to fight an incurable disease and the only witness to my efforts is often unable to let me know if I'm doing anything right. If you think I'm doing something, anything "right", please tell me so.

8   **Don't keep telling me about the latest miracle cure, research study or scientific article.** I hate this disease as well, but right now, my focus is on the person I love that is currently living with it, not on cures that may not be available for decades. A lot of these ideas may not ever come to fruition in time to help us and it just discourages me.

9   **You don't have to worry about saying or doing the right thing.** I don't always know what that is either. Please just keep trying. Don't avoid calling or coming over because you may be feeling uncomfortable or unsure. I feel that way too sometimes, and I'm here every day. We'll get through this, you and I, together.

10   **Please don't forget about me.** We're still here. We still love you. We still need and want you in our lives. There isn't any way you can interact with me that would be unwelcomed or wrong. Please just keep trying.

©2014, Mara Botonis, *"When Caring Takes Courage"*

CHAPTER 24

Legal, Medical and Financial Considerations

Despite the unpredictable course of the disease process when it comes to dementia (including Alzheimer's), there aren't many things that you can count on. One being that the more prepared you are for each contingency, the better able you'll be to meet the challenges that come your way. The second certainty is that you'll probably be in more than one situation where you'll wish you had answers or information before that moment.

Here are a few action items listed below that may be worth considering now to decrease the risk that you'll find yourself underprepared for a crisis or emergency in the future. The areas covered in this chapter include:

- ✓ Legal Matters
- ✓ Health and Medical Considerations
- ✓ Finances

Legal Matters

If your loved one has an attorney, make contact and advise them of your loved one's diagnosis. Also, check with the attorney and through all files available to determine if your loved one has executed any of the following instruments. If so, it is critical that you obtain and keep copies. Health care providers will often require copies of your loved one's medical record so be sure to have extra copies on hand.

Power of Attorney or (POA): There are several different types of Power or Attorney instruments that can be executed.

- A general POA-This allows an agent to act in all normal areas including purchasing or selling a property, signing contracts, and other legal actions.

- A springing POA: It derives its name because it "springs" into action only under certain conditions, such as incapacitation. How you are defining "incapacitated" should be clearly stated in the document.

- Durable POA: This instrument can either be ongoing or springing. It allows your loved one's designated agent's authority to continue to act on their behalf if your loved one becomes incapacitated.

Guardianship-A guardianship is initiated when a court appoints someone as the legal guardian for a person who is incapacitated in some way. In most cases involving guardianship, the elderly person is no longer able to make decisions about their own medical treatment, living conditions, dependents, and financial issues. Usually, a guardian is a family member or friend of the elderly person. If a friend or relative does not wish to become the person's legal guardian, a court-appointed guardian, or privately hired guardianship service can also serve. An elderly guardianship appointment is generally made if/when a court has determined that an elderly person is incompetent. The specific requirements for a court of law to legally declare your loved one incompetent can vary from jurisdiction to jurisdiction. As a general rule, however, is that whether a person is legally competent or not hinges on the ability to make informed and educated decisions about their personal affairs and the ability to meet his/her own physical needs.

Health and Medical Concerns

Complete the Biography Based Care® Alzheimer's/Dementia Patient Family Generated Health History Form: (this form is on pages 154-158): This tool has your loved one's medical history, current medical providers and contact information, current medications and insurance information all in one place. It is recommended that you keep three updated copies of this form; one in the home, one in your car and one with you. These days each medical provider or health care office seems to have their own new patient paperwork which can leave you constantly filling out the same information but on a different form every time. On these appointments or in the event of an emergency, having the Alzheimer's/Dementia Patient Family Generated Health History Form will save valuable time and prevent you from having to searching for medical provider contact information online, digging through wallets, etc.

- Advance Directives or Living Will: A legal document, signed by a competent person, to guide medical and health-care decisions (such as termination of life support or organ donation) in the event your loved one becomes incapable of making such decisions. Check with your primary care provider or legal advisor for more information about your specific situation.

- Do Not Resuscitate (or DNR): A do not resuscitate order can be part of an advance directive document or in some states it is a separate form. A properly executed DNR is to be followed if/when person's heart or breathing stops and they are unable to communicate their wishes to refuse treatment that could allow them to die. Laws regarding DNR orders vary by state, so local laws should be studied for specific requirements in your area.

Biography ❦ Based Care.

Alzheimer's/Dementia Patient Family Generated Health History Form

Full Name (first, middle, last)							
Date of Birth		Age		Marital Status		Religious Preference	
Veteran? Yes/No		Living Will or Advance Directive? Indicate "Yes" –or- "No". If "Yes", attach copy				Durable Power of Attorney? Indicate "Yes"- or- "No". If "Yes", attach copy	
Street Address							
City				State		Zip	
Allergies to any Food or Drug							

Social Security Number*			Medicare Number*		
Name of Insurance Company #1 (If Applicable)*		Group Number/ Policy Number		Insurance Company #1 Phone Number	
Name of Insurance Company #2 (If Applicable)*		Group Number/ Policy Number		Insurance Company #2 Phone Number	
Medicaid Case Number (If Applicable)		Medicaid Case Worker Name		Case Worker Phone Number	

Attach copies of cards. Healthcare providers will want copies of both front and back.

Primary Emergency Contact Name		Relationship to Patient	
Street Address			
City		State		Zip	
Cell Phone		Home Phone		Work or Alternate Phone	
Email Address			

Alternate Emergency Contact Name		Relationship to Patient	
Street Address			
City		State		Zip	
Cell Phone		Home Phone		Work or Alternate Phone	
Email Address			

Biography ❦ Based Care.

Alzheimer's/Dementia Patient Family Generated Health History Form

Full Name (first, middle, last)		Date of Birth	

Primary Care Physician		Office/Practice Name		
Street Address				
City		State	Zip	
Office Phone		Office Fax	After Hours/On Call Number	
Email Address				

Neurologist Name		Office/Practice Name		
Street Address				
City		State	Zip	
Office Phone		Office Fax	After Hours/On Call Number	
Email Address				

Specialty Physician Name		Office/Practice Name and area of specialty		
Street Address				
City		State	Zip	
Office Phone		Office Fax	After Hours/On Call Number	
Email Address				

Specialty Physician Name		Office/Practice Name and area of specialty		
Street Address				
City		State	Zip	
Office Phone		Office Fax	After Hours/On Call Number	
Email Address				

Biography ❧ Based Care®

Alzheimer's/Dementia Patient Family Generated Health History Form

Full Name (first, middle, last)		Date of Birth	

Pharmacy Name		Pharmacy Phone	
Street Address			
City		State	Zip
Pharmacy Fax		After Hours/On Call Number	
Email Address			

Medication Name	Strength (i.e. mg etc.)	Dosage (i.e 2 tablets, ½ tablet etc.)	Frequency (i.e 1 x daily, 2 x daily)

Biography ❦ Based Care®

Alzheimer's/Dementia Patient Family Generated Health History Form

Full Name (first, middle, last)		Date of Birth	

Past Medical History

Surgical Procedure	Date of Surgery	Performing Surgeon and Hospital/Outpatient Location

Significant Past Injuries or Medical Events	

Medical Diagnosis List	

Biography ❧ Based Care®
Alzheimer's/Dementia Patient Family Generated Health History Form

Full Name (first, middle, last)		Date of Birth	

Medical Problem List

Eyes			Ears		
Decreased vision	Yes	No	Decreased hearing	Yes	No
Infection/inflammation	Yes	No	Ringing/pain	Yes	No
Glasses	Yes	No	Hearing Aid(s)	Yes	No
Mouth			Nose		
Toothache/gum pain	Yes	No	Excess discharge	Yes	No
Difficulty chewing	Yes	No	Nosebleed	Yes	No
Dentures	Yes	No	Frequent congestion	Yes	No
Decreased sense of taste	Yes	No	Decreased sense of smell	Yes	No
Throat			Skin		
Soreness	Yes	No	Redness/rash	Yes	No
Difficulty swallowing	Yes	No	Open area(s)	Yes	No
Increased choking	Yes	No	Frequent bruising	Yes	No
Persistent cough/phlegm	Yes	No	Changes in hair or nails	Yes	No
Cardiac			Respiratory System		
High blood pressure	Yes	No	Frequent colds	Yes	No
Chest pain/tightness	Yes	No	Shortness of breath	Yes	No
Palpitations	Yes	No	Wheezing	Yes	No
Dizziness	Yes	No	Pain upon breathing	Yes	No
Vein trouble/leg pain	Yes	No	Difficulty breathing lying down	Yes	No
Swelling of ankles	Yes	No	Bluish lips or fingers/nails	Yes	No
Gastrointestinal/Endocrine			Nervous System		
Constipation	Yes	No	Frequent headache	Yes	No
Nausea/vomiting	Yes	No	Fits or convulsions	Yes	No
Diabetes	Yes	No	Change in sensation	Yes	No
Abdominal enlargement/distress	Yes	No	Poor coordination/balance	Yes	No
Heartburn/stomach pain	Yes	No	Tremors/twitching	Yes	No
Genitourinary			Muscle		
Incontinent of bowel or bladder	Yes	No	Stiff or swollen joints	Yes	No
Increased urination/urge	Yes	No	Muscle weakness	Yes	No
Pain or burning	Yes	No	Pain in joints	Yes	No
Change in sex drive	Yes	No	Decreased flexibility	Yes	No

Other:

_____

_____

_____

_____

Finances

Keep all listed financial information in a safe deposit box or lock box. If you already have a box, be sure that you know where the key is.

- ✓ Record your loved one's date of birth and Social Security number.
- ✓ Keep a copy of your loved one's driver's license, insurance and all other identification cards (even if it is not currently valid).
- ✓ Record the names and phone numbers of banking institutions and financial organizations where your loved one has accounts. Include numbers of checking & savings accounts, IRAs, CDs, investment accounts, etc.
- ✓ Look into having your name placed on checking & savings accounts and other income accounts so you can easily take over bill paying when the time comes.
- ✓ Check monthly balances on checking & savings accounts and be sure to reconcile the balances ensuring that bills haven't been forgotten or double paid and that there are no unauthorized charges or deductions on your loved one's account.
- ✓ Set up automatic electronic payment of recurring bills from known vendors to save time and reduce the risk of error.
- ✓ Record monthly income from Social Security, private pension funds, and all other sources of income.
- ✓ Make a list of any property or real estate holdings, car, boat or other vehicles that your loved one may own. Obtain titles of each.
- ✓ Make copies of health insurance, life insurance, and funeral policies.
- ✓ Keep copies of discharge and/or disability papers if your loved one was in the military.
- ✓ Keep a log with the date, time, organization, person, title and direct phone line/ email each time you speak with someone when applying for financial aid.

This may seem like an overwhelming list, and there are a lot of items that it would be nice for you to have. Start by gathering what you do have access to and then go online or call to order/request copies. In some cases, an in-person visit may be required to meet with a specific professional to obtain a document. Prioritize the medical and health related items and those you deem most important first and then work your way through the rest when you have the time and energy. This checklist is only a recommendation based on feedback from family caregivers. These are also tasks that you may choose to ask a well-meaning family member(s) to assist you with when appropriate. A trusted family member or friend can make appointments for you, print or download forms or do online research about various processes without you having to reveal sensitive financial or personal information.

CHAPTER 25

Overview of Home and Community Based Alzheimer's and Dementia Care Options

Knowing when to get more help with your loved ones care needs is only part of the challenge (see care planning tools in chapter 23 to help you determine how much help you may need) the other is determining where to get help in this day and age with more and more choices and options. Next, in Chapter 26 we'll share with you ways to make Alzheimer's care more affordable, but for now, let's start with what different levels of care are offered and then we'll work toward how to pay for them.

For this chapter we've divided the Alzheimer's/dementia care that's offered in most areas into two main categories, including the topics below;

1.) **Help While Your Loved One is Still At Home**: This section gives an overview of solutions that can be accessed from your home while your loved one still lives with you and includes:

✓ Adult Day Care
✓ Eldercare Sitter Services
✓ Live In Caregivers or Aides
✓ Home Care and Home Health Care
✓ Hospice and Palliative (Comfort) Care
✓ Respite (Short Term Stay) Care

2.) **Dementia (including Alzheimer's) Care Outside the Home**: When placement into a specialized care setting is optimal for your loved one's care.

✓ Adult Family or Group Homes
✓ Alzheimer's Facility
✓ Assisted Living
✓ Skilled Nursing
✓ Geriatric-Psychiatry (Geri-Psych) Facility

HELP WHILE YOUR LOVED ONE IS STILL AT HOME

Adult Day Care

Adult Day Care Centers provide care and companionship for seniors who need assistance or supervision typically during daytime hours, Monday through Friday, with recreational activities and noon-time meal usually included. Adult Day Care Centers (ADC's) operate under state specific guidelines, regulations, staffing and funding. Care levels provided and hours open may vary widely and some locations may even offer evening care and nursing support. Adult day care center rates vary and charges are not typically covered by Medicare, but financial assistance may be available through Alzheimer's charitable foundations Medicaid, the Older Americans Act, or The Veterans Administration (VA).

ADC's generally fall into two categories, a social and a health care model. Both of these are designed to offer at-home care partners alternative support and real relief for short periods of time. Accessing these types of programs may help delay memory care facility placement for your loved one by helping you avoid burnout.

The ADC social model provides social activities, meals, recreation and some basic health-related services. The ADC health care model offers more intensive health, therapeutic and social services for individuals with severe medical or behavioral challenges.

Seniors take part in the ADC program on a scheduled basis and often a pre-enrollment screening will be required to best determine if your loved one is a candidate for the program. Some ADC's will have a special Alzheimer's/dementia designation while others will focus on a more independent clientele that needs minimal supervision. Do ask questions up front to determine if the location(s) you are considering are truly staffed and trained to meet your loved one's special needs and be honest about any potential challenges the site may face in caring for your loved one. Disclosing a wandering risk or other behavior concerns early on will better help both your loved one and the ADC staff achieve better success in the long run or let you know early on that they are not equipped to safely accommodate them.

To find out more about the specific adult day care centers in your area, contact your Area Agency on Aging (AAA). The Eldercare Locator is another helpful resource that is a public service of the Administration on Aging at 1-800-677-1116 or on their website at www.eldercare.gov can help connect with these agencies.

The National Adult Day Services Association (NADSA) is also a good source of general information about adult day care centers and programs as well as guides you to resources in your location. The NADSA can be reached by calling the toll-free telephone number 1-877-745-1440 or by going to the website at www.nadsa.org.

Eldercare Sitter Services

Eldercare sitters are usually hired by families (versus agencies) to help ensure safety of and meet basic needs of persons with medical problems, such as patients who have suffered a stroke, traumatic brain injury, or have Alzheimer's disease or other forms of dementia. At times, hospitals, residential and care facilities may utilize these services (at the family's expense) when they feel a resident requires one on one or special supervision. Since sitters do not have to be licensed medical professionals, it is extremely important that you match their credentials and experience with your needs and ensure that you obtain references and a background check.

Costs vary, are usually billed hourly and may require a minimum number of hours per day. You may also be required to reimburse mileage for their trips on your behalf. Medicare and Medicaid typically do not pay for sitters, but some long-term care insurance policies or the Veteran's Administration (if an eligible beneficiary) might.

Check with your provider for more information on whether or not Sitter Services for your loved one are covered and are reimbursable expenses.

Most sitter services offer companionship, light housekeeping, errand running, shopping, and meal preparation. Some will have added training (e.g. they may also be a Certified Nurse's Aide –NAC) which, depending on your state's specific regulations, may allow them to assist with basic health needs such as taking vital signs or assisting with bathing for instance. Develop a written list that outlines duties and frequency of tasks you will want to be performed (see sample weekly care plan in Chapter 23). Clearly consider responsibilities upfront, so you know more about what you're looking for before you interview potential candidates.

It's important that a sitter knows what to do in an emergency and has the skill set and character that demonstrate you can trust them with your loved one. No screening process is foolproof. Below are some tips to help support you in the hiring process for eldercare sitters.

Let the individual or agency you choose to work with know that the care needed is for a person with Alzheimer's/dementia and that you'd like to employ an individual who, in addition to being compassionate and patient with person's diagnosed with the disease, also:

✓ Has 5+ years of experience caring for a person with Alzheimer's or dementia
✓ Is certified in dementia care by the Alzheimer's Association
✓ Maintains current CPR and First Aid certification
✓ Is legally allowed to work in the U.S. and has the all required documentation
✓ Has passed/will submit to a criminal background check
✓ Has 3-5 references of families they have previously worked for

Currently, there is not a comprehensive elder sitter service national directory produced by a government agency or non-profit group. However, the organizations below maintain lists of these services in many neighborhoods around the country and are free for families to use. Please note, however, that they refer to certain but not all elder care sitters in your area and typically feature those that have paid a fee to be listed on their materials and meet their specific criteria for inclusion.

Be diligent in asking for proof of healthcare credentials/certifications, background checks and references. For more information on senior sitter services in your area, contact: Sitter City at www.sittercity.com or call them at: 1-888-SIT-CITY or try www. care.com's eldercare advisor Helpline for a free consultation and referral at www.care. com or by calling them at 1-855-805-0711.

Live In Caregivers or Aides

A live-in care aid resides with the person they care for and is available to assist them during any time of the day or night. Live-in caregivers are usually given a room and expected to sleep over, and be "on call" if your loved one needs help during the night. A live-in caregiver has a caregiver partner who fills in so that he or she may have time off. If your loved one needs 24-hour "alert and awake" caregivers, then care is usually provided in two twelve-hour shifts with two caregivers, one of which is expected to be fully awake during his or her shift. The two person, round the clock model, is often recommended for someone who may be likely to wander, is up at night, needs toileting or assistance to and from the bathroom, exhibits frequent agitation or may be a danger to themselves or others.

Live-in elder caregiver costs can range and are generally paid weekly depending on duties performed, your loved one's care needs and level of supervision needed. You may also be required to reimburse mileage for their trips on your behalf. Medicare and Medicaid typically do not pay for live-in care, but some long-term care insurance policies or the Veteran's Administration (if an eligible beneficiary) might. Check with your insurance provider for more information on whether or not Sitter services for your loved one are covered or reimbursable expenses.

Most live in caregivers, like elder sitters, offer companionship, light housekeeping, running errands, shopping, and meal preparation. Some may have added training (e.g. they may also be a Certified Nurse's Aide –NAC) which depending on your state's specific regulations, may allow them to assist with basic health needs such as taking vital signs or assisting with bathing for instance. A written list outlining duties and frequency of tasks you will want to be performed is recommended for this position so that you might clearly discuss responsibilities upfront as you interview potential candidates.

It is important that the live-in caregiver knows what to do in an emergency and has the skill-set and character that demonstrates you can trust them with your loved one. Again, no screening process is foolproof. Below are some tips to help support you in the hiring process for a live-in caregiver or aide.

Let the individual or agency you choose to work with know that the care needed is for a person with Alzheimer's/dementia and that you'd like to employ a candidate who, in addition to being compassionate and patient with person's diagnosed with the disease, also:

- ✓ Has 5+ years of experience caring for a person with Alzheimer's or dementia
- ✓ Is certified in dementia care by the Alzheimer's Association
- ✓ Maintains current CPR and First Aid certification
- ✓ Is legally allowed to work in the U.S. and has the all required documentation
- ✓ Has passed/will submit to a criminal background check
- ✓ Has 3-5 references of families they have previously worked for

There is currently not a comprehensive national directory produced by a government agency or non-profit group for live-in caregivers. The following organizations, however, maintain lists of these services in many neighborhoods around the country and are free for families to use. Please note that they refer to certain but not all elder care sitters in your area and typically feature those that have paid a fee to be listed on their materials and meet their specific criteria for inclusion. Do be diligent in asking for proof of healthcare credentials and certifications, background checks, and references. For more information on senior sitter services in your area, contact: Home Care Assistance at www.homecareassistance.com or call them at 1-866-454-8346 (1-866-4-LiveIn) or www.homecareagencies.com for a directory of private duty and Medicare/Medicaid Certified Home Health agencies in your area.

Home Care

The terms "home care" and "home health care" are quite often used interchangeably to describe care provided in a private home versus a care facility. Often, persons with Alzheimer's/dementia also have a co-existing medical condition that impacts their physical health in addition to their cognitive impairment. These conditions may be chronic (such as difficulty swallowing) or situational (after a fall for instance), so the type of care needed varies based on the reason for the home care desired outcomes and projected length of home care service.

"Home care" services, also called, "companion care," are services that are largely non-medical in nature and refers to helping with household chores such as cleaning, shopping for and preparing meals, as well as assisting with some personal care like managing medications, minimal assistance with bathing, dressing and hygiene and even toileting. These services are usually paid for privately, and costs vary widely all over the nation. Check with your local providers for more information.

"Home health care" services must be ordered by a physician and provided by licensed and or trained medical personnel. In many cases, home health care services are required for those who have recently been discharged from a hospital or a skilled nursing facility but still require skilled medical care in their home for a period of time. Home health care may often be covered by Medicare/Medicaid, the Veteran's Administration (for eligible beneficiaries) and most long term care insurances provided their individual criteria is met, the care plan complies with their guidelines and is medically necessary. Home health care can include:

Skilled nursing care services such as management of feeding tubes, wound care, care of in-dwelling catheters or the administration of intravenous medications that must be provided or supervised by a licensed nurse, typically a Registered Nurse (RN).

- ✓ Physical therapy refers to rehabilitation services designed to restore and/ or maintain independence when a senior's physical strength has become compromised or diminished.
- ✓ Occupational therapy-works to improve or maintain independence in activities of daily living (such as dressing, bathing, grooming, etc.)
- ✓ Speech therapy-works to improve or maintain functions of speech, communication, swallowing, and language.

Home health agencies can provide these therapy services based on physician orders. The physician and therapy team will work together to determine what services are provided and the length of time each is required to regain maximum independence.

For more information on home care agencies in your area, visit the Medicare Home Health web page at:www.medicare.gov/homehealthcompare.com or call them at 1-800-633-4227.

Hospice and Palliative (Comfort) Care

Hospice and palliative or comfort care, are another example of terms that are often used interchangeably, but which are actually two different types of care.

Palliative care is specialized medical care for people with serious illnesses; it may not necessarily mean end of life care. Palliative care is focused on improving the quality of life through treatment or interventions designed to promote relief from the symptoms, pain, and the stress of a serious illness. Palliative care may be an appropriate option at any stage in a serious illness and can be provided along with curative treatment. This course of care is usually chosen once the person with dementia (or more likely their health care decision maker) decides to focus on comfort and quality of life.

For hospice, specific criteria must be met for a patient to qualify for benefits with a diagnosis of dementia. For a person with dementia (including Alzheimer's) to qualify for hospice care, the rule of thumb is generally that two doctors (usually your primary care physician and a physician that works with hospice) have to certify that the patient has a life-limiting illness and a life expectancy of six months or less. The life expectancy component was originally established by the Centers for Medicare and Medicaid Services (CMS), who notes on their website (www.medicare.gov) that "Unlike cancer, which typically follows a path of steady decline, dementia is much more difficult to predict. Patients with dementia may have periods of steady decline followed by an upswing, where they improve and do well for a time. For that reason, a special assessment tool was developed to help physicians identify when a dementia patient may benefit from hospice." Your loved one's physician may also consider medical complications, such as frequent hospitalizations recurrent infections (such as urinary tract infections, or blood infections) aspiration pneumonia (from choking on food or fluids) pressure sores on the skin and a refusal to eat. Ask your loved one's primary care physician more about when hospice may be appropriate for your loved one.

If a family desires comfort care for their loved one, who doesn't currently doesn't meet hospice eligibility criteria, there may be other options or "bridge" programs your local hospice provider offers. In these instances, make sure that your wishes are known to the physician and other health care providers regarding the intensity of treatments can help avoid unnecessary tests and procedures when weighing the outcome. Make sure all of your loved one's providers have copies of their Advanced Directives and (if applicable) Do Not Resuscitate (DNR) order.

Hospice and Palliative care may be covered by Medicare/Medicaid, the Veteran's Administration (for eligible beneficiaries) and most long term care insurances provided their individual criteria are met, and the care plan complies with their guidelines and is medically necessary.

For more information, contact the nonprofit National Hospice and Palliative Care Organization (NHPCO) at 1-703-837-1500 or visit their website at www.nhpco.org.

Respite (Short Term Stay) Care

Respite refers to a short-term care. It can provide temporary relief from the typical care routine that can allow the primary caregiver some down time while your loved one continues to receive care from qualified individuals and allows them the opportunity to have different experiences.

Respite care can be provided by paid staff, volunteers, or family or friends and can be offered at home, a community organization or a residential care center. The length of time respite care is provided can be for part of the day, during the evening, an entire overnight or for days or up to a couple of weeks. Respite care can be utilized occasionally, on a regular basis or just for emergency situations. There are many factors impacting your choice on which respite option may be best for you and your loved one including costs, availability/willingness of family or volunteers to help or your own scheduling and health constraints. In any case, it is not only okay to have systems in place to provide care for your loved one when needed, but it is also highly recommended.

Many families have found themselves in an emergency situation requiring immediate action that was less than ideal because they failed to plan ahead for a time when their loved one's primary caregiver may be temporarily unable to meet care needs.

A barrier often heard from family members about voluntarily accessing respite care solutions in non-emergent situations were feelings of guilt. Many expressed guilt that their loved one doesn't get a break from dementia, so they don't deserve a break from caregiving. Another argument against respite was the concern that other's wouldn't know how to care for a loved one as well as they do along with the worry that their loved one would feel abandoned or angry with them. These are real and understandable feelings. In an emergency situation, such as the primary caregiver's hospitalization or illness, it is easier to set these feelings aside to cope with the crisis at hand, but along with those very valid feelings and concerns, please take a moment to consider these thoughts as well.

In home-respite care can support the primary care partner in being more effective by:

□ Creating time to take care of errands that you can't or prefer not to do with your loved one in tow, thus avoiding the need to put them in situations that may be over-stimulating such as shopping, pharmacy, or other errands/outings or time for things that you need to do on your own (i.e. your own medical appointments, getting your haircut, etc.).

□ Offering the care partner a chance to spend time with friends and family, or to just relax and take some time to experience something other than dementia-related pursuits. This brief reprieve can help renew your spirit and reenergize you for the increasingly difficult tasks ahead. You are in a marathon race against the disease that is dementia (including Alzheimer's), and the pace you keep can have a significant impact on the quality of your run. Just like a runner needs enough water and nutrition and physical training to run their best race, a care partner needs to ensure adequate breaks to be their emotional, physical and overall best self. You may not think you deserve this time for yourself, but that's not true! You need to take this time for your loved one. It will make you a better, more compassionate, patient and loving caregiver.

There are also benefits for your loved one as well. Respite can offer those with Alzheimer's/ dementia, a controlled break from their routine in the way that you determine is most beneficial for them. Factors in choosing the right respite solution and setting can be made a little easier when you consider these factors in your decision making:

✓ Will this allow my loved one to interact with others having similar experiences?
✓ Will he/she be able to spend time in a safe, supportive environment that is not over-stimulating while being different enough to facilitate interest?
✓ Will my loved one be presented with the opportunity to participate in enjoyable activities designed to match personal abilities and needs?
✓ Is the person(s) responsible while I'm away adequately trained to handle the needs of people with Alzheimer's/dementia and my loved one specifically?

In-home respite care services are provided at home to assist the caregiver and the person with dementia. Informal respite care is when family members, or friends, are willing to help. Even for just a few hours, to give the primary care partner time to run errands, get some sleep or just to take a short break. Caregivers should keep in mind these people who have previously offered to help. Make note of when others are available before you need them to make planning ahead a little easier.

For more information on in-home respite care providers, in your area, contact:

✓ ARCH –The National Respite Locator Service, at 1-919-490-5577, or visit their website at www.arch.org.
✓ The Eldercare Locator, a public service of the Administration on Aging at 1-800-677-1116 or visit their website at www.eldercare.gov
✓ The Alzheimer's Association's Care Finder at 1-800-272-3900 or search their website at www.alz.org/carefinder for a provider listing
✓ A Place for Mom at 1-866-321-7634 or visit their website http://www. aplaceformom.com/
✓ Caring.com at 1-800- 952-6650 or visit them online at https://www.caring.com/

Alzheimer's Care Outside the Home

Before we begin the portion of this chapter that explores care outside the home, let's take moment to consider the many criteria that you might likely want to evaluate as you consider which provider is the best fit for you.

On the following pages, you'll find the Biography Based Care ® Alzheimer's Care Comparison Score Sheet, which is a tool to will help you evaluate and compare different residential options for your loved one based on widespread industry standards and accepted guidelines for Alzheimer's/dementia care. It is recommended that you bring this care comparison score sheet with you as you visit these communities and compare the score you give them to the information you gather from their brochure, consumer reviews, online research, and word of mouth.

The score sheet offers recommended questions for you to ask as well as an easy to use scoring system to support you in objectively comparing g providers based upon criteria such:

- ✓ Affordability
- ✓ Appearance-Physical Plant/Décor
- ✓ Dementia Expertise
- ✓ Dining
- ✓ Family Friendly Programs and Opportunities to Collaborate on Care
- ✓ Family Testimonials (what are current clients saying about this organization?)
- ✓ Room Size/type
- ✓ Secured/safe environment
- ✓ Staffing
- ✓ State Health Department Survey/Audit Results

Additionally, the score sheet has lots of room for to joy down your overall opinions and experiences regarding the providers you are considering. This is a great tool for multiple decision makers to use to better communicate with one another what they did or didn't like about a particular provider's program or services and why.

Biography ♥ Based Care®
Alzheimer's/Dementia Care Comparison Score Sheet

Rating System: Use one column per provider. Enter a numeric score in the space provided rating up to 3 providers in each of the criteria to consider. Rate the providers be awarding them a numeric score from 1-10, with 1 being the lowest and 10 being the highest. Base your rating on your opinion of how satisfied or dissatisfied you are with what you've learned from each organization as you complete your research.

Criteria To Consider	Option #1: Organization Name: — Scoring 1-10: 0-4: Below Expectations, 5-7: Meets Expectations, 8-10: Above Expectations, Or Mark: N/A	Option #2: Organization Name: — Scoring 1-10: 0-4: Below Expectations, 5-7: Meets Expectations, 8-10: Above Expectations, Or Mark: N/A	Option #3: Organization Name: — Scoring 1-10: 0-4: Below Expectations, 5-7: Meets Expectations, 8-10: Above Expectations, Or Mark: N/A
Affordability: -Are there options that adjust the rate as your loved ones care needs increase or decrease over time? -Does this organization accept State/Medicaid pay in the event private funds may run out? Will they direct bill your long term care insurance, VA or other insurance company? -What is their discharge policy regarding residents who are no longer able to pay their bill?			
Appearance: -Is the layout of the community easy to navigate? Do the hallways lead residents back to public areas? -Are color, lighting, noise level and décor pleasant and calming? -Does it appear clean? Odor free? -Furniture and amenities in good condition and working order? -Are residents encouraged to bring in familiar items and decorate according to their preferences? -Does the environment offer areas that residents can access with or without staff to enjoy their hobbies and interests?			
Dementia Expertise: -Do the caregivers have specialized training in effectively communicating with and caring for residents with Alzheimer's/dementia? -What training has occurred for specific behaviors and interventions? -Are ongoing educational programs provided to staff by their own corporation or other outside agencies regularly? -Does the orientation/performance review process for care staff include skill demonstration handling behaviors and interacting effectively with Alzheimer's/dementia residents?			

Dining:
- Are meal times flexible?
- What kind of supervision is provided during meal times?
- How much assistance and cueing is offered to those that require it?
- Are meals "dementia friendly" i.e. lots of finger foods, smaller portions, and 5-6 smaller meals offered versus 3 larger ones?
- Are snacks and nutritional supplements (i.e. shakes) available 24 hours per day to offer to residents?
- Are special diets accommodated?
- What is their policy related to both care and discharge for a person is no longer able or willing to eat food orally?

Family Friendly:
-- Are visiting hours generous and meet your needs for access to your loved one?
- Are there adequate spaces for private visits with your loved one around the community or in their room?
- Can your loved one participate in outings from the facility with you (If medically able and appropriate)?
- Are there opportunities for you to participate alongside your loved one in activities as well as socialize with other families regularly?
- Is there a family council or committee that meets regularly, is attended by administration representatives and allows family members a forum to advocate for their loved one as well as give input regarding the enhancement overall operations?
- What systems do they have in place to resolve family complaints or concerns?

Family Testimonials:
- Ask to be contacted by at least 3 family members of current residents that you can speak to about their experiences
- Search the community or organization as well as parent company online to review feedback and customer reviews
- What are the most common complaints received? How have they been addressed?

Room Type/Size:
- Do the residents have adequate privacy for bathing, toileting and hygiene?
- Are residents encouraged to personalize their space?
- If shared accommodations, what systems in place to best pair up roommates, resolve conflict?

	Total Score Option 1: ___/100 0-49: Below Expectations 50-79: Meets Expectations 80-100: Above Expectations	Total Score Option 2: ___/100 0-49: Below Expectations 50-79: Meets Expectations 80-100: Above Expectations	Total Score Option 3: ___/100 0-49: Below Expectations 50-79: Meets Expectations 80-100: Above Expectations
Secure Environment: -Are all exterior doors and exits alarmed and monitored to ensure the safety of residents who are wander? -Do residents wear a wander guard or personal alarm triggered when accessing doors outside or other potentially unsafe areas? -Are outdoor patios and walking areas easily accessible to residents yet enclosed to prevent wandering away from the community? -How do staff members respond to an elopement or wandering incident? Have they ever had an elopement? What was the outcome?			
Staffing: -What type of licensure is required for key members of the care team? Is the Director a licensed nurse? -How many hours is the community staffed with a licensed nurse (RN or LPN)? - Have staff members been screened with state/national background checks? -How is stuffing adjusted aside from sheer # of residents to ensure that as care needs increase staff/resident ratios are adequate? -Do staff seem accessible to residents? -Are staff and resident interactions unhurried, patient, kind and appropriate (note body language, word choices and tone of voice while staff are interacting with residents)			
Survey Results: -By law, communities or organizations surveyed or reviewed by the state must have available for public viewing their recent results. Ask to read their most recent annual survey -Are the citations in a category that did not cause grave harm or negative outcomes? -Did the community file their plan of correction to address the issues identified in the citation? -Were their additional state visits triggered by complaints? How were those resolved? -Did the community ever face monetary penalties or temporary bans of new resident admissions based upon their state survey findings?			
Totals: Add the total points for each option vertically to arrive at an overall numeric score for each option.			

Biography ♥ Based Care®

Alzheimer's/Dementia Care Comparison Score Sheet

Additional Notes and Overall Impressions:		
Option #1: Organization Name: Contact Person: Phone:		
Option #2: Organization Name: Contact Person: Phone:		
Option #3: Organization Name: Contact Person: Phone:		

Adult Family or Group Homes

Group or Adult Family Homes (AFH's) provide care to a group of people with similar disabilities within a residence, often an actual home. It is extremely important to do your homework when considering this level of care, as homes, staff training, and capability vary widely as do individual state regulations governing the type of care that can be provided in this setting. Check with your state for any violations and recent survey results, the status of their license, complaints, and history. You will also want to tour, ask for references of current and past family members and check with the Better Business Bureau and online for consumer reviews and customer feedback.

Group or AFH care is generally not covered by Medicare. Medicaid, Long Term Care Insurance Policies and/or the Veteran's Administration (for eligible beneficiaries) may offer some coverage if qualifying criteria is met. Check with your policy holder or government program administrator to learn more about whether your loved one can access these benefits.

There is no national database of AFH's, but your yellow pages, online directory, or Area Agency on Aging office will be a good place to get local listings.

Alzheimer's Care Communities in General

Look for designations like "memory care" or dementia-capable" when doing research on Alzheimer's/dementia care communities, and be sure to use the Alzheimer's/Dementia Care Comparison Score Card on pages 173-176 to ask the questions that will help you find the best fit for your loved one.

For a FREE list of Alzheimer's specific care providers in your area, contact:

- ✓ The Eldercare Locator, a public service of the Administration on Aging at 1-800-677-1116 or visit their website at www.eldercare.gov
- ✓ The Alzheimer's Association's Care Finder at 1-800-272-3900 or search their website at www.alz.org/carefinder for a provider listing
- ✓ A Place for Mom at 1-866-321-7634 or visit their website http://www.

aplaceformom.com/

✓ Caring.com at 1-800-952-6650 or visit them online at https://www.caring.com/

Assisted Living

Assisted Living Facilities (ALF's) are residential communities for seniors who want or need help with some of the activities of daily living such as bathing, dressing, grooming, medications management and toileting for example. Most assisted living communities offer different types of living arrangements from a simple room without private bathroom to studio, one bedroom, and larger apartments and even cottage homes on their campuses. Some come with full or mini-kitchenettes that can be single occupied or shared with a spouse or another resident. Typically, there are common areas for shared dining, activities, and hosting guests.

Each state has its own unique specific licensing guidelines and operating regulations that dictate things such as the level of care that can be provided, staffing levels and other considerations. In general, meals, recreational activities, transportation, housekeeping, laundry services, with staff available 24 hours per day, etc. are some common offerings in assisted living facilities across the country.

Assisted living communities, unless specifically noted may not be equipped to handle middle to late stage Alzheimer's/dementia. Some assisted living communities offer secured Alzheimer's areas for those that exit seek and/or offer specially trained staff, Alzheimer's adapted activities and increased staffing and supervision in their "general population" for those residents. Each state has its own licensing regulations for assisted living, so you'll want to learn more about what services are provided in your area.

Assisted living is usually paid for privately. Some communities will accept Medicaid residents and long-term care insurance as well as Veteran's Aid and Attendance beneficiaries. Check with each assisted living provider you are considering to learn more about to the payment methods they accept.

Assisted living costs vary widely depending upon both, type of living arrangement and level of care provided. In some cases, a move in fee, deposit or first month's rent will be required before admission.

For more information on Alzheimer's/memory care specific Assisted Living providers in your area, contact:

- ✓ The Eldercare Locator, a public service of the Administration on Aging at 1-800-677-1116 or visit their website at www.eldercare.gov
- ✓ The Alzheimer's Association's Care Finder at 1-800-272-3900 or search their website at www.alz.org/carefinder for a provider listing
- ✓ A Place for Mom at 1-866-321-7634 or visit their website http://www.aplaceformom.com/
- ✓ Caring.com at 1-800- 952-6650 or visit them online at https://www.caring.com/

Skilled Nursing Facility (SNF) or commonly called Nursing Homes

A nursing home is usually one of the highest levels of care for older adults outside of a hospital. A physician supervises each patient's care and a nurse/other medical professional is normally on site 24-hours a day. Allied health professionals, such as speech, occupational or physical therapists, are also commonly available. Having the medical team, on-site allows for the delivery of medical procedures and therapies that are not possible in other more independent housing settings. Nursing homes provide both a higher level of short-term medical and rehabilitative care and longer-term custodial care. Custodial care at this level can include total assistance getting in and out of bed, support with feeding, bathing, and dressing. Medical care at this level may include the supervised use of oxygen, administration of intravenous medications and tube feedings. Rehabilitative care in a skilled nursing setting may include physical, occupational, speech and/or respiratory therapy. State licensing requirements for SNF levels vary, so be sure to inquire at each facility you are considering to learn more about the scope of services and staffing they offer.

According to the Centers for Medicare and Medicaid Services (CMS) website (www. medicare.gov) Medicare will pay some nursing home costs for eligible beneficiaries who meet criteria and require skilled nursing or rehabilitation services. To learn more about Medicare payment for skilled nursing home costs, contact the State Health

Insurance Assistance Program (SHIP) in your state. Medicaid will pay for skilled care provided in a Medicaid-certified nursing homes/skilled nursing facilities. For more information about Medicaid, call the SHIP for your State or call your State's Medicaid office. The SHIP phone number for each state can be found online or in your telephone directory.

For more information on SNF's in your area, contact:

- ✓ Medicare by phone at 1-800-MEDICARE (1-800-633-4227) or visit their website: www.medicare.gov/nursinghomecompare/search.
- ✓ The Eldercare Locator, a public service of the Administration on Aging at 1-800-677-1116 or visit their website at www.eldercare.gov
- ✓ The Alzheimer's Association's Care Finder at 1-800-272-3900 or search their website at www.alz.org/carefinder for a provider listing
- ✓ A Place for Mom at 1-866-321-7634 or visit their website http://www. aplaceformom.com/
- ✓ Caring.com at 1-800- 952-6650 or visit them online at https://www.caring.com/

Geriatric In-Patient Psychiatry (Geri-Psych) Facility

Geriatric psychiatry, (also known as Geri-psychiatry) deals with the study, prevention, and treatment of mental disorders in older adults. A Geri-psych facility is often a specific unit or floor of a hospital that is geared toward inpatient care for someone in acute need of geriatric psychiatry services. A Geri-psych unit is often used for emergency placement of a person who is deemed a danger to themselves or others. Persons who are classified as posing this risk after an evaluation by a trained professional can be admitted to a Geri-psych unit involuntarily while efforts are made to resolve any underlying medical issues, adjust medications or implement behavioral interventions. If you think your loved one may be a danger to themselves or others (including you), IMMEDIATELY dial 911. First responders can intervene and assess the current risk and make a referral to other mental health professionals if needed.

Geri-psych services can be costly if paid privately. However, care is often reimbursable by Medicare, Medicaid or your private insurance if pre-authorization and admission criteria are met.

Geri-psych units/programs are located in or affiliated with acute care hospitals, so the best way to determine if your area has a Geri-psych program is to contact your local hospital. Currently, there is not a national directory or website with a database for this level of care. Contact your local acute care hospitals to determine if they offer this specialized program.

CHAPTER 26

Financial Solutions for Affording Care in Today's Economy

Now that you know more about the levels of care and options both in and outside the home that support the daily needs of a person with Alzheimer's/dementia, the next logical question is likely to be, "how can I afford help?" With healthcare costs continuing to rise and the added financial stress felt by many families, affording help for care of a person with Alzheimer's/dementia may feel out of reach. This chapter is designed to acquaint you with a few of the various methods of paying for home or facility based care services. These programs each have different qualifying criteria and guidelines and in each case, Included in this chapter, are website and/or contact number(s) to connect you directly with the program administrators so you may learn more about your potential eligibility or to gather more information.

NOTE: Information about the programs on the following pages does not constitute an endorsement or recommendation to use any of these programs and in no way should be considered financial advice. You and your family, accountant, attorney or trusted advisors may be the best group to decide what financial solutions are most beneficial for your particular situation.

In alphabetical order, in this chapter, you'll find a brief overview of:

- ✓ Bridge Loans (Senior Care Bridge Loan)
- ✓ Life Insurance (surrender of an in-effect policy for cash value for needed healthcare)
- ✓ Long Term Care Insurance

✓ Medicaid
✓ Medicare
✓ Respite or Short Term Stay Programs and Scholarships
✓ Reverse Mortgage Home Loans
✓ Scholarships
✓ Shared or Semi-Private Suites (how to save up to 40% off single occupant rates)
✓ Tax Deductible Health Care
✓ Veteran's Administration Aid and Attendance Program

* Information contained herein was gleaned directly from websites and other printed material from the organization(s) mentioned directly. Eligibility criteria and benefit amounts are updated often, so be sure to contact each organization directly for current guidelines.

Bridge Loan (Senior Care Bridge Loan)

There is a loan product that is specifically designed as a Senior Care Bridge Loan. The "Elderlife Line of Credit" from Elderlife Financial is an example of this kind of loan and is designed to help seniors and their families cover the costs associated with assisted living, home care or skilled nursing on a short term basis. A line of credit for care is offered to qualified borrowers. Payments are made directly from the loan to the care provider. At no point do the borrowers take possession of the funds. What is different about this type of loan/line of credit is that up to six co-borrowers can apply which allows multiple family members or friends to share in the cost of paying for a loved one's care. The Elderlife Financial Line of Credit is an unsecured loan, meaning co-borrowers are not required to put up a home or vehicle as collateral. A fairly good credit score is required for approval. These loans also have a very fast approval process. Individuals can be approved in as little as one to three days though typically more time would be needed if there are co-borrowers.

This type of loan is typically earmarked to specifically cover costs associated with senior care such as: paying for move in fees or buy in costs to enter a care community, to pay for room/board and care while awaiting the sale of a home or start of Veteran's

Aid and Attendance benefits for example.

Alzheimer's/dementia care are included in what is considered needed care provided they contact Elder Life Financial directly (to get pre-authorization) by calling them at 1-888-828-4500 or visit their website at www.elderlifefinancial.com.

Life Insurance Cash Out (surrender an in-effect policy for cash value for needed healthcare)

Some types of life insurance policies can be a means to raise funds for care. Check with your loved one's life insurance provider to see if you may be able to borrow from the policy's cash value or receive part of the policy's face value (known as a viatical loan) which would be paid off upon the person's death.

Some life insurance policies also offer accelerated death benefits, meaning that some of the insurance benefits may be paid before death if the insured person is not expected to live (beyond a predetermined number of months) due to a terminal illness. The payout may run as high as 90 to 95 percent of the policy's face value. Check with your life insurance carrier directly and be sure to have a written copy of your policy for reference as you determine whether or not this may be an option in your specific situation.

You can learn more about viatical loans by visiting www.viatical.org or calling them at 1-800-973-8258.

Long-Term Care Insurance

Long-Term Care Insurance (LTCI) refers to private insurance health care policies that can cover a portion of eligible healthcare related expenses (such as home healthcare, assisted living, adult daycare, or nursing home) and are typically purchased BEFORE you need it because health status is taken into consideration. It is usually recommended that LTCI is purchased at a younger age when premiums are lower because many carriers may exclude certain pre-existing conditions.

LTCI policies are often used to cover expenses that are not generally covered by private insurance, Medicare, or Medicaid. Some plans offer the option to purchase in-home care in addition to assisted living, adult day care, respite care, nursing home care, and hospice care. The plans and their specific exclusions and eligible coverage amounts vary widely depending on the policy.

If you know your loved one has long term care insurance, obtain a written copy of the policy and notify your insurance provider that your loved one has Alzheimer's and you'd like to learn more about what care options are available. If you aren't sure if you have LTCI, start with your current insurance agent to see if they have any information for you and check bank records for recurring monthly premium payments that may identify the LCTI carrier.

A resource to answer general questions is the "American Association for Long-Term Care Insurance" (AALTCI). They can be reached by phone at: 1-818- 597-3227 or visit their website at: www.aaltci.org.

Medicare and Medicaid

Medicaid and Medicare are two very different governmental programs that provide medical and health-related services to specific groups of people in the United States. They are both managed by the Centers for Medicare and Medicaid Services (CMS), which is a division of the U.S. Department of Health and Human Services. Information in the following section was obtained from www.medicaid.gov.

Medicaid

Medicaid can provide medical and care service for eligible low-income seniors. If your loved one is financially and medically qualified, Medicaid will pay for nearly all of their long-term care. Medicaid would send payments directly to the participating health care providers for services provided to Medicaid recipients. Each state sets specific Medicaid guidelines. The program meant to assist people with low incomes, but eligibility also depends on meeting other requirements such as disability status, the age of the applicant, and personal assets being below a set level. If eligible, Medicaid can help cover the costs of routine and emergency health care (such as inpatient hospital services, outpatient hospital services, physician services, nursing facility services, home health care for persons eligible for skilled-nursing services, laboratory, x-ray, diagnostic services, prescribed drugs and prosthetic devices, optometrist services and eyeglasses, transportation, rehabilitation and physical therapy services, home and community-based care for certain persons with chronic impairments).

Each state has its' own application and approval process, and the guidelines are updated yearly. The eligibility criteria for the Medicaid program follows federal guidelines (below) that may help you determine potential eligibility. For more information, call the Centers for Medicaid and Medicare Services (CMS) at: 1-800-772-1213 or visit them on their website at www.medicaid.gov.

To be eligible for Medicaid, one must be financially qualified; but to be eligible for Medicaid's long-term care services, one must also be medically qualified. Each state considers the following three factors for Medicaid's long-term care services:

✓ Medical Necessity for Health Care Services – an individual must be unable to care for him/ herself and requires assistance with the activities of daily living or need ongoing supervision.
✓ Income Level – You will want to check with your local program to learn more about the specific acceptance criteria in your area.
✓ Assets and Resources – currently, the "Countable Resources" limits, which exclude the car and home of primary residence, vary.

Medicare

Medicare is a Federal health insurance program that pays for hospital and medical care for individuals over 65 years old, (or in certain cases, younger persons with qualifying disabilities). The program consists of two main parts for hospital and medical insurance (Part A and Part B) and two additional parts that provide flexibility and prescription drugs (Part C and Part D). Check the front of your loved one's Medicare card to see which Medicare coverage they have. Your loved one may also have a Medicare Supplement that is paid for privately to cover the co-pay on Medicare Eligible services.

Each policy varies widely, so call your private insurance carrier for more information about any Medicare Supplemental your loved one may have through their company. For more information on Medicare, you can call the Centers for Medicaid and Medicare Services (CMS) at: 1-800-633-4227 or visit their website at: www.medicare.gov. In some cases, Medicare MAY pay for in-home care services. Below is a brief overview of the Medicare program per their website:

Medicare Part A, or Hospital Insurance (HI), helps pay for hospital stays, which includes meals, supplies, testing, and a semi-private room. Part A also pays for home health care such as physical, occupational, and speech therapy that is provided on a part-time basis and deemed medically necessary. Care is typically provided in a skilled nursing facility, provided pre-admission criteria is met (most often used after a hospital stay) as well as certain medical equipment for the aged and disabled such as walkers and wheelchairs. Part A is generally available without having to pay a monthly premium since payroll taxes are used to cover these costs.

Medicare Part B is also called Supplementary Medical Insurance (SMI). It helps pay for medically necessary physician visits, outpatient hospital visits, home health care costs, and other services for the aged and disabled. For example, Part B covers durable medical equipment (canes, walkers, scooters, wheelchairs, etc.), X-rays, laboratory and diagnostic tests, some ambulance transportation for example. Part B requires a monthly premium and patients must meet an annual deductible amount before coverage actually begins. Enrollment in Part B is voluntary so again, check the front of your loved one's Medicare Card to see if your loved one has opted to pay for this additional coverage.

Medicare Part C (Medicare Advantage Plans or Medicare + Choice) allow users to design a custom plan that can be more closely aligned with their medical needs. These plans enlist private insurance companies to provide some of the coverage, but details vary based on the program and eligibility for the patient. Some Advantage Plans team with Health Maintenance Organizations (HMOs) or preferred provider organizations (PPOs) to provide preventive health care or specialist services. Others focus on patients with special needs such as diabetes.

Medicare Part D (often called prescription drug coverage) is administered by one of several private insurance companies, each offering a plan with different costs and lists of drugs that are covered. Participation in Part D requires payment of a premium and a deductible.

Respite or Short Term Stays (in assisted living or skilled nursing homes)

Many assisted living communities and skilled nursing facilities have Respite or Short Term Stay programs that allow families to obtain care for their loved one on a short-term basis (usually the length of stay is between 5 to 30 days) without a long-term or permanent move.

Typically a fully furnished room or apartment is made available after a pre-admission nursing evaluation conducted by the care community you choose to ensure that your loved one fits their admission criteria. A short term move-in can occur rather quickly, often within a day or two of your initial inquiry. There are state specific requirements that care providers must comply with and as a result, you'll likely need to obtain a health history, physical and current doctor's orders from your physician.

Check with your local assisted living and skilled nursing providers to determine which ones offer short term or respite stays, what their specific daily rates are and any specific admission requirements that they may have.

For a list of Alzheimer's care respite providers in your area, contact:

- ✓ The Eldercare Locator, a public service of the Administration on Aging at 1-800-677-1116 or visit their website at www.eldercare.gov
- ✓ The Alzheimer's Association's Care Finder at 1-800-272-3900 or search their website at www.alz.org/carefinder for a provider listing
- ✓ A Place for Mom at 1-866-321-7634 or visit their website http://www.aplaceformom.com/
- ✓ Caring.com at 1-800- 952-6650 or visit them online at https://www.caring.com/

Reverse Mortgage Home Loan

A reverse mortgage is a loan product that may be an option for eligible homeowners. Eligibility ages and criteria vary depending on the lender. The collateral for a reverse mortgage is the home's equity. Typically, a reverse mortgage home loan doesn't need to be repaid until approximately six months after either the homeowner passes way, the home is sold, or the last surviving homeowner leaves the residence.

While the eligibility requirements vary, most lenders that offer a reverse mortgage have the same requirements as those for the Federal Housing Administration's Home Equity Conversion Mortgage (HECM). For more information, contact a reverse mortgage specialist at your local financial institution or contact the U.S. Department of Housing and Urban Development (HUD) at: 1-800- 225-5342 or log onto the HUD website to read more about reverse mortgages at: www portal.hud.gov.

To be considered eligible for HECM reverse mortgage, homeowners must:

- ✓ Own their home either outright or have enough equity built up to qualify.
- ✓ The mortgage balance must be low enough to be paid off completely by the proceeds of the reverse mortgage at loan closing.
- ✓ Applicants must reside in the home.
- ✓ Applicants cannot be delinquent on any federal debts.
- ✓ HECM reverse mortgage applicants will need to receive free or low-cost counseling from an HECM counselor to ensure that they understand the terms of the loan.

Scholarships

Some chapters of the Alzheimer's Association have a set aside a portion of their annual funding which has been earmarked for Respite or Short Term Stay scholarships offering emergency relief for caregivers of persons with Alzheimer's/dementia by paying for all or a portion of their daily care for a set period. Although the Alzheimer's Association is a national organization, the individual chapters administer their respite program differently. Contact the Alzheimer's Association helpline (operating 24 hours a day, 7 days per week) at: 1-312-335-8700 or visit their website at: www.alz.org to get the phone number of the Alzheimer's Association chapter nearest you and speak with them directly to find out if they have a respite scholarship program, what the eligibility criteria are and how to apply.

Shared or Semi-Private Suites (how to save up to 40% off single occupant rates)

Many assisted living communities and skilled nursing facilities that offer Memory (Alzheimer's) Care have a shared or semi-private (also referred to as companion living) suites option that would pair them with a roommate.

Having a roommate can decrease the cost of care up to 40% or more off of the cost of private room rates. Most families would prefer their loved one has their own room or apartment, but this may be a helpful option for you if it means the difference between being able to afford care.

In some situations, the companionship offered in a roommate situation may help your loved one enjoy needed social interaction in a way that is more comfortable for them than participating in group activities. Most communities that offer these type of living arrangements for persons with Alzheimer's/dementia are also familiar with resolving any disagreements that may potentially arise over who's things are who's or conflict related to disorientation.

There are many other factors aside from financial savings to consider, however, and some of them may include asking these questions of yourself, the community you are considering and your physician:

- ✓ How does my loved one do interacting with other people one on one?
- ✓ How does the community determine whom my loved one will "room" with?
- ✓ What alternatives are available if my loved one and their roommate are just not compatible?
- ✓ How much/little time might my loved one spend in their room versus in common areas participating in activities or meals?
- ✓ What effect might a roommate have on my loved one's sleeping habits and

daily routines?

Check with your local assisted living and skilled nursing providers to determine if they offer shared or semi-private suites. Be sure to ask what their specific daily rates are for your loved one's room and their care.

For a list of Alzheimer's care providers in your area that offer shared or semi-private suites contact:

- ✓ The Eldercare Locator, a public service of the Administration on Aging at 1-800-677-1116 or visit their website at www.eldercare.gov
- ✓ The Alzheimer's Association's Care Finder at 1-800-272-3900 or search their website at www.alz.org/carefinder for a provider listing
- ✓ A Place for Mom at 1-866-321-7634 or visit their website http://www.aplaceformom.com/
- ✓ Caring.com at 1-800- 952-6650 or visit them online at https://www.caring.com/

Tax Deductible Health Care

Many families may not know that in addition to the programs mentioned throughout this chapter that can help make care costs more affordable on the front end, there are also programs that help you deduct from your income or receive credit for the money you have spent on senior care on your taxes on the back end.

Most costs associated with home, medical and assisted living care, prescription drugs and medical equipment and supplies are usually considered tax-deductible through various state and federal tax credits. However, available tax credits and deductions vary widely based on a variety of factors. Contact your accountant, tax professional or the Internal Revenue Service Directly at: 1-800-829-1040 or visit their website at: www.irs.gov.

Below are a few tax terms related to tax credits and deductions for elder care that you may want to become more familiar with.

Dependent Status? One of the first things you may want to identify is whether your loved one's taxes should be filed separately or if it better to claimed them as a dependent. To claim a loved one as a dependent:

☐ The tax filer must have provided at least half of the dependent's financial support for the year or, if more than one family member is pitching in to cover 50% of the dependent's living expenses, then the family would pick just one person to claim the loved one in need of care as a dependent.

☐ The dependent must be a relative of or have lived with the tax filer for one full calendar year.

Tax Credits and Deductions for Elderly Dependents -it is recommended you use one of the many tax calculators available online or contact your accountant/tax professional to help you determine the best course. Also referred to as the Child and Dependent Care Credit; is a tax credit for families who incur expenses to cover the costs of home care or adult day care of a loved one, so that they can work. Many states have their own version of the Federal Child and Dependent Care Credit Program so be sure to ask your accountant about this.

Medical and Dental Expense Deductions - Medical and dental expenses can be deducted in some cases. It is recommended you use one of the many tax calculators available online or contact your accountant/tax professional to help you determine if any of your loved one's medical or dental expenses meet deduction criteria.

Veteran's Aid and Attendance benefits

Aid and Attendance is a benefit paid by Veterans Affairs (VA) to veterans, veteran spouses or their surviving spouses who need financial help for in–home care, to pay for an assisted living facility or a nursing home.

The monthly award benefit for eligible recipients can range and may be contingent upon meeting the following requirements per www.va.gov:

☐ If the veteran or the veteran's surviving spouse was discharged from a branch of the United States Armed Forces under conditions that were not dishonorable AND served at least one day (did not have to be served in combat) during wartime.

☐ If the veteran or veteran's spouse is already eligible for the VA basic pension.

☐ The aid of another person is needed in order to perform personal functions required in everyday living, such as bathing, feeding, dressing, toileting, adjusting prosthetic devices, or protecting himself/herself from the hazards of his/her daily environment; or the claimant is bedridden (e.g. his/her disability or disabilities require that he/she remain in bed apart from any prescribed course of convalescence or treatment); the claimant is in a nursing home due to mental or physical incapacity; or the claimant is blind, or so nearly blind as to have corrected visual acuity of 5/200 or less, in both eyes, or concentric contraction of the visual field to five degrees or less.

☐ The claimant's countable family income must be below a yearly limit set by law.

The veteran or surviving spouse will need to gather the following VA Forms (Forms can be found at http://www.va.gov/vaforms/) before applying for benefits:

- ✓ Discharge or Separation Documents (DD 214).
- ✓ VA Form 21-22 if represented by a Veteran's Service Organization or 21-22a if an individual is acting as the claimant's representative.
- ✓ Form 21-4142: Authorization and Consent to Release Information to the Department of Veterans Affairs.
- ✓ Letter from the claimant's attending physician VDVA Form 10.
- ✓ Physician Statement, VA Form 21-2680 or Nursing Home Statement, VA Form 21-0779
- ✓ Medical Expenses incurred, VA Form 21-8416.
- ✓ In addition to the VA forms, an applicant will need to gather the following documents:
- ✓ Marriage Certificate and Death Certificate (Surviving Spouses only).

✓ Asset Information (bank account statements, etc.)
✓ Verification of Income (social security award letter and statements from pensions, IRAs, annuities, etc.)
✓ Proof of Medical Premiums (Insurance Statements, Medication or Medical bills that are not reimbursed by Medicaid or Medicare).
✓ Voided Check for Aid and Attendance if Direct Deposit is desired.

Contact the VA directly for more information on potential eligibility at Veteran's Affairs: 1–800–827–1000 or you can apply online at https://www.ebenefits.va.gov/.

CHAPTER 27

Free Resources for Family Care Partners

A lot of care partners report feeling equal parts isolated and overwhelmed during journey with a loved one through dementia (including Alzheimer's). However, there are many, many more resources available to uplift, educate and inspire us.

In this chapter, I'm sharing some of my favorite ways for families to access free and helpful resources right from home. The best part is not only are they free, but you can access them when you get a moment. It doesn't matter if you haven't had time to take a shower today or are reading this at 1:30 in the morning, these things are here for you when you have time and space to explore them. Also, you don't need to find care for your loved one so you can leave home--these things come to you, on your time.

Please know that this is by no means meant to a comprehensive list of every free tool that's available, and there are more and more free resources are popping up all the time. Each website, organization, expert, blog or online group has a little different philosophy, culture and tone. Be sure to "try a few on" so that you can see which offer the best fit for you.

Here are some of our favorite family care partner "freebies":

Activity Engagement Tools

☐ **Adult Coloring Pages**
- http://www.coloringpagesforadult.com/
- http://www.coloringprintables.net/adult-coloring-pages.html

☐ **Classic Television** (sorted by series and decade)
http://retrovision.tv/all/

☐ **Classic Movies** (sorted alphabetically and by title)
http://www.bnwmovies.com/

☐ **Exercises for Seniors** (5 minute video classes and handouts)
http://seniorexercisesonline.com/

☐ **Nostalgic Trivia Questions For Seniors**
http://www.triviacountry.com/371-American-trivia-questions.html

☐ **Printable Memory Games**
http://www.memozor.com/memory-game-online-free/
printable-memory-games/memory-for-adult

☐ **Vintage Radio Broadcasts** (sorted by decade, show and genre)
  • http://www.companionradio.com/crwp/golden-ages/
  • http://radiolovers.com/

☐ **Reminiscing Articles and Photos** (sorted by decade and area of interest)
www.reminisce.com (note: there are free posts on their website)

Apps
☐ **Care Zone** (from AARP)
☐ **Care Buddy** (from the Alzheimer's Association)

Booklets
☐ **Advance Care Planning Booklet** from www.usa.gov. Call 1-719-295-2675 for print copies or download your free copies of this and 34 other Alzheimer's related publications from: http://publications.usa.gov/USAPubs.php?PubID=2307
☐ **Alzheimer's Care Booklet** from www.usa.gov. Call 1-719-295-2675 for print copies or download your free copies of this and 34 other Alzheimer's related publications from: http://www.publications.usa.gov/USAPubs.php/Alzheimerscare

□ **Caring for a Person with Alzheimer's Disease Guide** from the National Institute of Health. Call 1-800-222-2225 for print copies or download of this and over 50 other Alzheimer's related booklets from: https://www.nia.nih.gov/alzheimers/publication/caring-person-alzheimers-disease/about-guide **Managing Stress for the Caregiver** booklet from the Bright Focus Foundation. For a print copy, call them at 1-800-437-2423 or download your own from: http://www.brightfocus.org/sites/default/files/caringcaregiver_stress.pdf

Blogs

□ **Alzheimer's.net by A Place for Mom:**
http://www.alzheimers.net/blog/

□ **Alzheimer's Association Blog:**
http://blog.alz.org/

□ **Alzheimer's Disease Expert by Mayo Clinic:**
http://www.mayoclinic.org/diseases-conditions/alzheimers-disease/expert-blog/CON-20023871

□ **Alzheimer's Disease and Dementia by about.com:**
http://alzheimers.about.com/

□ **Alzheimer's Reading Room by Bob DeMarco:**
http://www.alzheimersreadingroom.com/

□ **Alzheimer's Speaks by Lori La Bey:**
https://alzheimersspeaks.wordpress.com/

□ **Family Caregiver's Blog by the National Family Caregiver Alliance:**
https://www.caregiver.org/blog

□ **Minding our Elders by Carol Bradley Bursack:**
http://www.mindingoureldersblogs.com/

☐ **Tales of Alzheimer's and Caregiving by Maria Shriver:**
http://mariashriver.com/blog/category/alzheimers-and-caregiving/

☐ **The Long and Winding Road Journey Through Alzheimer's by Ann Napoletan:**
http://alzjourney.com/

☐ **Patient with Dementia Symptoms by Truthful Loving Kindness:**
http://truthfulkindness.com/

☐ **The Caregiver's Voice Blog by Brenda Avadian, MA**
http://thecaregiversvoice.com/blog/

Care Planning

☐ **Advance Care Planning** booklet from www.usa.gov. Call 1-719-295-2675 for print copies or download your free copies of this and 34 other Alzheimer's related publications from:
http://publications.usa.gov/USAPubs.php?PubID=2307

☐ **Caregiver Toolbox** collection of booklets from the U.S. Department of Veteran's Affairs. Call 1-800-827-1000 to order print copies or, download your own from :
http://www.caregiver.va.gov/toolbox/index.asp

☐ **End of Life: Helping with Comfort and Care** booklet from www.usa.gov. Call 1-719-295-2675 for print copies or download your free copies of this and 34 other Alzheimer's related publications from:
http://publications.usa.gov/USAPubs.php?PubID=2219

☐ **Your Guide to Choosing a Nursing Home or Other Long-Term Care Booklet** from the U.S. Department of Health and Human Services. Call 1-719-295-2675 for print copies of download from http://publications.usa.gov/USAPubs.php?PubID=5337

Clinical Trials/Research Information

☐ **The Alzheimer's Association's Trial Match:**
http://www.alz.org/research/clinical_trials/find_clinical_trials_trialmatch.asp

☐ **Clinicaltrials.gov:**
https://www.clinicaltrials.gov/

Diagnosis and Symptoms Tools

☐ **Alzheimer's Disease Booklet** from the Alzheimer's Association -call for print copies 1-800-272-3900 or download from http://www.alz.org/alzheimers_disease_publications.asp

☐ **Living Well with Dementia** booklet from the Alzheimer's Association. Call for a free print copy or download your own from their website at: http://www.alz.org/documents/mndak/alz_living_well_workbook_2011v2_web.pdf

e-Newsletters

☐ **Alzheimers.net's "Inspirational Newsletter" e-Newsletter:**
http://www.alzheimers.net/inspirational-newsletter/

☐ **Alzheimer's and Dementia Weekly's "Alzheimer's Weekly" e-Newsletter:**
http://www.alzheimersweekly.com/

☐ **Alzheimer's Association's "Alzheimer's Weekly News" e-Newsletter:**
http://www.alz.org/apps/email_signup.asp

☐ **Alzheimer's Foundation of America's "AFA e-Newsletter":**
http://www.alzfdn.org/Publications/enewsletter.html

☐ **Alzheimer's Reading Room's Weekly E-Newsletter:**
http://www.alzheimersreadingroom.com/

☐ **Caregiver.com's "Today's Caregiver" e-Newsletter:** http://www.caregiver.com/caregiver_newsletter/index.htm

☐ **Caring.com's "Steps and Stages" and/or "Caring Suggests" e-Newsletters:** https://www.caring.com/newsletters

☐ **Fisher Center For Alzheimer's Research Foundation's e-Newsletter:** http://www.alzinfo.org/news/e-newsletter/

☐ **Mayo Clinic's "Alzheimer's Caregiving" e-Newsletter:** https://newslettersignup.mayoclinic.com/?fn=203

☐ **Teepa Snow's "Positive Approach Care" e-Newsletter:** http://teepasnow.com/

☐ **UsAgainstAlzheimer's "Weekly News" e-Newsletter:** http://www.usagainstalzheimers.org/content/contact-us

Facebook Support Groups

☐ **Alzheimer's and Dementia Caregivers Support Group**
☐ **Caregivers and the Elder Care Community**
☐ **Dementia Spouse Group**
☐ **Memory People**
☐ **UsAgainstAlzheimer's Support Group**

Helplines

☐ **The Alzheimer's Association:** 1-800-272-3900
☐ **The Alzheimer's Foundation of America:** 1-866-232-8484

Magazines (Printed copies you can order by mail and online versions)

☐ **Care Quarterly** by the Alzheimer's Foundation of America. Call 1-866-232-8484 to order your print copy or download the electronic version of the magazine here: http://www.alzfdn.org/subscription2.html

Money Matters

☐ **The Family Medical Leave Act (FMLA) Guide** from the Department of Labor. Call 1-866-487-9243 to order your free print copy, or download from http://

www.dol.gov/whd/fmla/employeeguide.pdf

☐ **Medicare Basics: A Guide for Families and Friends People with Medicare** booklet from www.usa.gov. Call 1-719-295-2675 for print copies of download from http://publications.usa.gov/USAPubs.php?PubID=6039

☐ **Money Matter booklet from the Alzheimer's Association.** Call 1-800-272-3900 for a free print copy or download your own from their website at: http://www.alz.org/national/documents/brochure_moneymatters.pdf

Radio on-Demand Programs

☐ **Alzheimer's Speaks Radio:**
http://www.blogtalkradio.com/alzheimersspeaks

Webinars

☐ **Communicating Effectively with your Doctor** from the National Family Caregiver's Alliance on-demand webinar, go here to watch: **http://app. brainshark.com/NFCA/vu?pi=zJWzeuhgcz2mqgz0**

☐ **EssentiALZ series from the Alzheimer's Association** on-demand webinars, go here to watch:
http://training.alz.org/

☐ **Family Caregiver Alliance Alzheimer's** caregiving series on-demand webinars, go here to watch: https://www.caregiver.org/caregiving-webinars

Websites:

☐ **A Place for Mom:** http://www.aplaceformom.com/

☐ **AARP Webplace:** www.aarp.org
Administration for Community Living: http://www.acl.gov/
Alz.Live: http://alzlive.com/

☐ **Alzheimer's Association (National):** www.alz.org

☐ **Alzheimer's Bookstore:** www.alzheimersbooks.com

☐ **Alzheimers.com – Caregiving Resource:** www.alzheimers.com

☐ **Alzheimer's Companion Magazine:** www.alzheimerscompanion.com

☐ **Alzheimer's Disease Education and Referral Center:** www.alzheimers.org

- ☐ **Alzheimer's Family Organization:** www.alzheimersfamily.org
- ☐ **ALZwell Caregiver Support:** www.alzwell.com
- ☐ **American Health Assistance Foundation/Alzheimer's Family Relief Program:** www.ahaf.org
- ☐ **Caring.com:** https://www.caring.com/
- ☐ **Center for Medicare & Medicaid Services (CMS): www.medicare.gov**
- ☐ **Dementia Action Alliance:** http://daanow.org/
- ☐ **Empowering Caregivers:** www.care-givers.com
- ☐ **The Family Caregiver Alliance:** www.caregiver.org
- ☐ **John's Hopkins Memory Center:** http://www.hopkinsmedicine.org/psychiatry/specialty_areas/memory_center
- ☐ **National Academy of Elder Law Attorneys** (NAELA): www.naela.org
- ☐ **National Alliance for Caregiving:** www.caregiving.org
- ☐ **National Family Caregivers Association:** www.nfcacares.org
- ☐ **National Institute on Aging (NIA): www.nih.gov/nia**
- ☐ **Mayo Clinic:** http://www.mayoclinic.org/diseases-conditions/alzheimers-disease/
- ☐ **Science Daily (link to the latest research news): www.sciencedaily.com**
- ☐ **UsAgainstAlzheimer's:** http://www.usagainstalzheimers.org/

Videos

- ☐ **The Alzheimer's Project by HBO Films:**
  http://www.hbo.com/alzheimers/caregivers.html

- ☐ **CCAL's "Advancing Person Centered Care video:**
  http://www.ccal.org/person-centered-matters-video/

- ☐ **Sandy's Story with Dr. Sanjay Gupta on CNN:**
  http://www.cnn.com/2015/10/12/health/alzheimers-sandys-story/index.html

- ☐ **Teepa Snow's Tips:**
  https://www.youtube.com/user/teepasnow

☐ **Virtual Dementia Tour:**
http://www.alzheimersweekly.com/2013/01/experience-12-minutes-in-alzheimers-on.html

CHAPTER 28

Healing the Hurt: What to Do When Your Family Feels Fractured

You've watched so many hours of Oprah, Dr. Phil and reconciliatory themed Hallmark Channel movies that you feel like an amateur family therapist. You've apologized for the times it was your fault, and turned the other cheek while trying to forget the times it wasn't. You've reached out so many times that you feel like one arm is actually longer than the other.

You've tried to put the past in the past, manage your own hurt feelings and release regrets in the name of mending fences, only to have your feelings hurt anew with each interaction or lack thereof. If your family is like most families, the lifetime of shared experiences you've had and memories you've created together have run the gamut from fulfilling to frustrating and everything in between.

Having a relationship in need of repair with someone you care about is tough enough under "normal" circumstances. Adding the impact of dementia (including Alzheimer's) to an already fragile family dynamic, it's enough to make any of us head straight into a good long "ugly cry" as soon as we're alone.

Sometimes it can feel like a hopeless situation that isn't likely to improve. However, despite all of this hurt filled history, at the end of the day, you miss this person, you love this person and you wish things were better between you. But how can it be when it truly feels like you've already tried everything you can do to make it better?

The first thing we need to do is objectively self-reflect on that last part (the part where despite all of the justifiable reasons where we get to be the hero of our own narrative who has endured a legitimate or perceived wrong) we actually and honestly look at things a little differently.

Sometimes giving up can feel a lot easier than giving it another try. But, if there hasn't been any truly physically or emotionally abusive behavior (which is inexcusable), then maybe one of the ideas below can give you another way to fight for a better relationship with someone you don't want to give up on.

Here are some ways we can work to improve our relationships:

☐ Identify how you want the relationship to grow or improve. Putting it down on paper and looking at these wishes can help you focus on the future instead of what's already occurred and help ground you when you're in the heat of the moment.

☐ Ask yourself honestly whether your past actions (and future ones too-before you act/speak on them) support or decrease the chances that the relationship will improve and grow the ways you hope for. Sometimes, whether we want to admit it or not, our behavior can actually be contributing to a delay on the path to a full reconciliation.

☐ Forgive them. Forgive yourself. Maybe in this case you weren't the one that was "wrong" maybe in this case you are doing everything "right"…but we both know it hasn't always been this way. We've all done or said things at one time in our life or another that we'd like to take back or do differently. This person is no different. They may regret their behavior, but not know how to "fix" it, or they may be incapable of understanding the hurt they are causing. We may never know why some people act the way they do. What we do know is that we aren't flawless people, so it isn't very fair to expect that level of perfection in others. It isn't our job to measure others with our own yard stick. How short might we "measure" up if others do that to us?

☐ Own it, apologize for it and avoid doing it again. You can't undo your mistake, but you can lessen the negative impact if you are truly honest in your self-reflection. If you are genuine in your self-awareness and authentic in your apology about what you did to contribute to the strife and if you are sincere in your desire to avoid repeating the same, you'll be making a great step toward growing both yourself and the relationship.

☐ Talk to them, not about them. I know you need to talk this difficult situation out, to vent about it, to process what's happened because you're hurt and the other person may not be very open to a healthy conversation right now. It's not only OK, but maybe therapeutic to talk to others about things that are bothering you, but that should also be tempered with equal parts talking about what you can do to make it better and reaching out to the person directly. Too many times the need to process what we're feeling with others can turn into an all-out recruitment effort to create allies in a war you don't even want to fight. Lay down the weapons that gossip or harmful words can become and avoid enlisting others in your anger.

☐ Don't add insult to injury. Avoid fanning the flame and widening the divide between you by adding new reasons to be angry at each other. If your relationship is currently in an awkward or uncomfortable place, the first thing you can do to repair it is, not make things worse. Practice "if/then" scenarios before they occur so you can prepare a more positive response. If you know this person is likely to say or do something that bothers you, think about how you might respond differently next time so you can help diffuse versus escalate the situation. This is a lot easier to do "in the moment" if you've given it some thought beforehand.

☐ Avoid snarky social media posts. I'm not sure anyone involved in a difficult family dynamic has changed their behavior, had an epiphany or evolved their way of thinking all of a sudden because of a sassy Facebook cartoon or a status update describing the thinly disguised offenses of "some people." This goes back to that honest earlier evaluation about whether our own actions are helping or hurting the healing process. If you need to vent, do it privately with a trusted confident, away from the eyes and ears of everyone you know.

☐ Is it more important to be "right" or be together? Having a better relationship with this person will likely involve some compromises, and maybe more on your part than you'd like. Maybe the "right" thing would be that your sibling helps with the day to day care of your parent as much as you do, but if that's not happening, then maybe it's time to be OK with seeing them when they do show up-because having them around a little, is better than not ever seeing them at all. Work on what will create more quality time together. That could mean making then feel more comfortable around you by avoiding blame, resentful remarks, or re-airing of past problems and painful moments when you do see them again. Getting closer may actually look a lot like letting some things go.

Days become weeks, weeks give way to months and soon the time you've been estranged accumulates faster than either of you would want. Sometimes we are so sure that we are right, that we are willing to live at that virtual address of above reproach until we realize we will forever occupy that space all alone. Waiting for the other person to make the first move, or change or "see things my way" may be a long and lonely vigil, and chances are, the other person is thinking the same thing about you.

Forgiveness, hope, love, and family are values many of us hold dear. If possible, err on the side that pursues each of these.

But, it's also OK to trust yourself. Know when to say when. This is the tough one. Only you know when the hurt this relationship causes eclipses the healthy aspects of being in each other's lives. Only you know when it's time to stop trying.

We all hope that never happens. I hope you don't let it happen until you try the ideas above at least one more time.

CHAPTER 29

Maintaining Your Role When Others Oversee Direct Care

The decision to arrange for others to participate in meeting your loved one's daily care needs is never an easy one. By and large the most common concern I've heard from families who were considering facility placement or the hiring of in-home primary caregivers may surprise you.

Often the primary barrier to obtaining increased care didn't come down to overcoming feelings of guilt, or even financial considerations…instead it was something harder to articulate and even harder to overcome. There was an inexplicable sense that after their loved one moved into a care community, the gradual erosion of the relationship with their loved one would suddenly be accelerated to the point that any hope of further connection would forever be lost. The fear that what remained of a once powerful bond would slip past the point of recognition to be retrieved again only in frozen moments captured in old photos or relegated to the occasional retelling of family stories. Those feelings are real, those feelings are completely understandable.

Even when you are the face your loved one sees most often, the disease process means that recognition does fade. It's only natural to worry that when your loved one lives away from home in a different environment or is cared for by other people that this fading away may happen more quickly. However, ensuring that your loved one receives adequate care to meet their increasing needs is likely your overriding priority, even if that comes with the potential for some additional hurt and grief.

Below are some tips about how to feel connected and stay an important part of your loved one's life no matter where they are or who is helping with their care:

☐ Create space to share your stories. You most likely sought care outside the home or hired professional care givers to come in because they possess an expertise with Alzheimer's/dementia that you feel would benefit your loved one. But, their expertise is with the *disease* not with the *person*. There is no one else who knows your loved one better than you and you've had a front row seat with which to view and be an important part of their life story, their biography. Your voice is needed to communicate your loved one's history, preferences, likes and dislikes when they are no longer able to do so. This information is critical in assisting the care team in meeting daily emotional and physical needs.

☐ Feel good about giving advice. It's okay to share with others your caregiving successes, routines, and preferences. You've been at this a while and as anyone with any experience in Alzheimer's/dementia care knows, what worked one day can be totally ineffective the next. The more ideas and approaches you can share with your new caregiving team, the more choices they will have when needed as different situations arise. They may already know about the disease process, but they are just learning about your loved one, so your tips and suggestions should be met with appreciative ears as they work to establish their own relationships and schedules with your family member.

☐ Consider what is most meaningful and then share your own needs. Be honest about what you need from this experience. Most primary caregivers are excellent at communicating what they feel their loved one's needs are, but many have gone so long without making their own well-being a priority that they may not be accustomed to thinking about what they need. Think about the times during the day that you feel most connected to your loved one, the times or activities that bring you the most joy or satisfaction. Let the caregiving team know that you'd still like to be the one who washes your Mother's hair, feeds your Dad Sunday dinner, shaves your Husband's familiar face or play your Wife's favorite songs from the days you courted. Letting the care team know that this means a lot to you can help them create space and time for those experiences to continue. It is an all-around win-win situation as it's enriching for your loved one, meaningful for you and a great chance for the caregiving team to take a little break.

☐ Ask often to be included and involved. When it comes to coping with the effects that Alzheimer's/dementia has on family life, each person is different. Even members of the same family may choose to handle the changes in their loved one and their shared relationship very differently. Many caregivers are taught to let the family member(s) set the tone for how much or how little involvement they'd like to have in their loved one's daily life. Let the care team know the different ways you'd like to participate. Are their opportunities to join a family council or support group? Do they need volunteers to help with special events and activities? Are they in need of any activity or other supplies that you could help with? Are there any special projects that you could assist with such as creating an edible garden or bird houses that would benefit all? Sometimes being a part of the community, family groups or helping the care team can help fill the emotional void when visits with your loved one end with you wanting more of an emotional connection.

☐ Set regular care conferences and meetings. Most care providers have minimum expectations set by the state or other regulatory agencies as to the frequency and type of formal communications with family members regarding the scope of care, current challenges, and changes in the care plan. Be sure to make it a point to schedule these regularly (most are monthly, quarterly or when there has been a significant change in condition) and ask for copies of the care plan or written notes for your reference. These meetings (different than the kind of calls that report an incident, injury or emergency) are an important time for everyone who is a stake holder in your loved one's care to come together and collaborate on the best possible care solutions as your loved one's needs change.

☐ Articulate your communication needs. Unless you ask for something different, many providers will contact you according to their policy. When there has been an injury, incident, emergency or regularly scheduled care conference. Whether they care for multiple patients, or just one, the shift of a caregiver is full of unpredictable surprises and constant demands for their time and attention. You may need to make it a point to prepare them for the kind of communication you want and need ahead of time. For example, write down your questions and let them know you'd like to check back with them in a day or so when they've had a chance to research the answers. This technique is particularly helpful when your questions are around things like medications, recent lab results, new physician orders, challenging behaviors, eating and sleeping patterns, weight gain/loss or even interaction with others and level of enjoyment with recreational programs. They will not only need to pull your loved one's medical record/chart, but will also likely need to consult with others to give you the most accurate information. You may also want to let them know in advance the kinds of information that you'll be asking for most often. For example, do you want to know how your loved one has been sleeping? Did they participate in any activities? When they are almost out of their medication if you want to be the one to refill it? Each time a physician or consultant has been contacted? Letting the care team know what most important to you can help support them in responding to your queries more quickly.

☐ Schedule your visits and create a new routine. It can be overwhelming to adjust to the difference between being "on call" 24 hours a day, every day as the primary caregiver, to all of a sudden having a choice between how you help and how often you help with your loved one's care. Many families have asked me over the years, after placing a loved one in a community, which course of action is best. Should they visit often or stay away completely in the early stage of the transition to help their loved one adjust? The short answer is neither. Every situation is different and requires some flexibility as both you and your loved one get used to new routines. You should know that there is no "right" or "wrong" way to get through this phase. But, a little planning can make it a lot easier. Get a calendar out and take a moment to think about what you want the first few weeks of this transition to look like. Schedule time to be together during the hours that are most meaningful or important (meals, activities, or doctor's appointments). This is where that old saying about quality time versus quantity time really comes into play. Visiting every day, three times a week or setting goals around the number of your visits is not nearly as important as scheduling based upon the quality of your visits. Consider what time is best for your loved one. Would you being there during meals be a distraction or a help for example. Maybe they have most of their energy in the morning but are more anxious and fearful in the afternoon. When would your loved one most need your visit? When would you be more likely to get the most out of your time together? When would your presence be most helpful in accomplishing care goals? When would you be best able to contribute to your loved one's life enrichment? And last, but not least, when would you most enjoy your time together?

☐ Give yourself permission to visit or participate in your loved one's care on your own terms without fear of judgment internally or from others. Some days will be harder than others, some decisions and duties you'll need to carry out will be tougher than you thought while others will be surprisingly rewarding just when you need it most. It's okay to embark on this in your own way. That's the only way to do it.

☐ **_No one_** but **_you_** knows what it feels like to love this person, to lose parts of this person to Alzheimer's/dementia and to suit up every day even when it takes everything you've got to continue to be there for someone who may not even remember who you are. What matters is that you remember who they are. You remember all of the great, funny, sweet, silly and sad moments that make up your shared history. However you choose to honor and protect that is up to you and only you. Don't let your idea, real or imagined of other's expectations dictate the course of a journey that only you alone know how to travel. Trust yourself. Step back when it hurts too much, come closer when you are strong enough and be there when you are able, so you can savor every moment that unexpectedly brings back that familiar smile, that well-known twinkle in the eye or the touch of a hand that reminds you of that which will never be forgotten, that Alzheimer's disease may have _changed_ the love you shared, but it will never, can never, and doesn't have the power to ever, erase it.

CHAPTER 30

The Generous Gift of a Great Goodbye

It would be easier for us to give in to anticipatory grief, to get lost in the sadness that our loved one's impending physical absence will soon bring after all of the months we spent losing them cognitively due to Alzheimer's. It would be a lot easier to let the constant tears welling up flow freely into unrestrained sobs. When it was time for us to say good-bye to my Grandfather, we took a different approach.

We didn't want to wait to have his "Celebration of Life" after he passed; instead we wanted him to be included.

I'm proud of us as a family for doing what he taught us to do through his lifelong example of putting others first. On Grandpa's last day with us, we didn't spend those precious hours fulfilling our own needs around the fellowship of our shared impending grief instead we coordinated wordlessly to make sure whatever time he had left with us, was the best it could be.

My Grandpa's last day was filled with loving whispers from his wife, joyful stories of his children, the recollections of his grandkids, and the sounds of his favorite music. His last day was filled with the reassuring touch of his loved ones, the constant sensation of warm blankets, and the calming scent of the lavender plants so prevalent on the Northwest peninsula where he lived and surrounded by a love so strong that I'm convinced that though wholly unresponsive, on some level, he could still feel it.

We fell apart many days after that one and we still do, but we didn't do it that day, we wouldn't let ourselves do that on his last day. On that day, we gave him the only thing we could, the only thing that he might have needed or wanted in that moment;

we gave him The Generous Gift of a GREAT Good-bye.

Saying goodbye to a loved one before they pass is never easy, but here are 5 ways to make it a little better for them.

- ☐ Sounds: Fill their room with their favorite music, people (or recorded messages from family and friends), and happy stories about their life and legacy. Think about what your loved one would most want to hear.

- ☐ Sights: Even if they are not opening their eyes much, or at all, fill their room with favorite and uplifting sights. Pictures, posters, flowers, balloon bouquets, familiar memorabilia and faces. Try to mask the grimace of grief on your face with loving looks when you are near them in case they open their eyes.

- ☐ Touch: Bring in soft textiles, and cuddly things to hug or touch. Warm bedding and bedclothes in the dryer to offer comfort (ask staff to help with this if your loved one's last days are occurring at an in-patient setting such as hospital, nursing home or hospice. Offer the reassurance of your physical touch frequently if it does not cause pain. Kisses on their forehead, gentle hand massages and reassuring pats on the arm can let your loved one know that they are not alone.

- ☐ Scents: Use aromatherapy to create calm or evoke familiar favorites through lotions, room or linen spray. Soaps and lotions with favorite scents can be used for personal care and smells of favorite foods even if they are not eating may bring a sense of home.

- ☐ Taste: At this stage, your loved one may have stopped eating by mouth long ago. To prevent the lips from drying, offer a moistened swab with lemon or flavored lip balm to sooth the skin and encourage swallowing between breaths.

Your loved one's life story unfolded with a unique combination of experiences page by page or decade by decade while living, their passing will likely be just as personal and specific to them. Every family copes with the end stages of the disease process differently and there is no "right" or "wrong" way to say good-bye.

It's perfectly normal to have a range of feelings right now. The nature of your relationship with your loved one (before and after onset of symptoms), the type and length of care giving support you were providing, the level of physical and emotional stress you are under, family dynamics and overall fear and worry can all impact how you are thinking and feeling at this time.

Some family care partners report feeling such a deep sense of sadness while others share a sense of relief that their loved one's suffering may be coming to an end. Give yourself space to feel what you are feeling without self-criticism or internal judgements.

Hospice support can help you plan out what you'd like these last few days/hours to be like, so that you have some support in planning during this very emotional and difficult time. If your loved one is not receiving Hospice care, consider reaching out to your family, care giver support groups and spiritual community for fellowship.

Appendix

I.

Recommended Reading List

A Heart Full of GEMS (Someone my child loves has dementia)
By Rev. Linn Possell, Teepa Snow

A Personal Guide to Living with Progressive Memory Loss
By Sandy Burgener & Prudence Twigg

A Pocket Guide for the Alzheimer's Caregiver
By Daniel C. Potts M.D. and Ellen Woodward Potts

Ageless Outings – Summary of Ageless Outings – Destination Planning Chart &
Appendix of Destinations Listed Alphabetically
By Maureen Wells

Alzheimer's: A Caregiver's Guide and Sourcebook
By Howard Gruetzner

Alzheimer's Early Stages: First Steps for Family, Friends and Caregivers
By Daniel Kuhn, MSW

Alzheimer's from the Inside Out
By Richard Taylor PhD

Before I Forget: Love, Hope, Help, and Acceptance in Our Fight Against Alzheimer's
By B. Smith, Dan Gasby, Michael Shnayerson

Being My Mom's Mom
By Loretta Veney

Can't We Talk about Something More Pleasant? A Memoir
By Roz Chast

Caring For Your Parents (The Complete AARP Guide)
By Hugh Delehanty and Elinor Ginzler

Changes in Decision-Making Capacity in Older Adults: Assessment and Intervention
By Sara Honn Qualls, Ph.D. and Michael A Smyer

Chicken Soup for the Soul: Living with Alzheimer's & Other Dementias: 101 Stories of Caregiving, Coping, and Compassion
By Amy Newmark and Angela Timashenka Geiger

Coach Broyles' Playbook for Alzheimer's Caregivers: A Practical Tips Guide
By Frank Broyles

Come Back Early Today: A Memoir of Love, Alzheimer's and Joy
By Marie Marley PhD

Creating Environments of Support: A Handbook for Dementia Responsive Design
By Sarah Campernel & William Brummett, William Brummett Architects

Creating Moments of Joy for the Person with Alzheimer's or Dementia: A Journal for Caregivers (4th ed.)
Edited by Jolene Brackey

Doing Things: A Guide to Programming Activities for Persons with Alzheimer's Disease and Related Disorders
By Jitka Zgola

Elder Rage, or Take My Father... Please!: How to Survive Caring for Aging Parents
By Jacqueline Marcell

Finding Joy In Alzheimer's: New Hope for Caregivers
by Marie Marley Ph.D. and Daniel C. Potts M.D.

From the Corner Office to Alzheimer's
By Michael Ellenbogen

Jan's Story: Love Lost to the Long Goodbye of Alzheimer's
By Barry Peterson

Keeping Busy: A Handbook of Activities for Persons with Dementia
By James Dowling

Learning to Speak Alzheimer's: A Groundbreaking Approach for Everyone Dealing with the Disease
By Joanne Koenig Coste

Love in the Land of Dementia: Finding Hope in the Caregiver's Journey
By Deborah Shouse

Mayo Clinic on Alzheimer's Disease
By Mayo Clinic and Ronald Peterson

On Pluto: Inside the Mind of Alzheimer's
By Greg O'Brien

Seasons of Caring: Meditations for Alzheimer's and Dementia Caregivers
By ClergyAgainstAlzheimer's Network and Jade C. Angelica

Slow Dancing with a Stranger: Lost and Found in the Age of Alzheimer's
By Meryl Comer

Staying Afloat in a Sea of Forgetfulness
By Gary Joseph LeBlanc

Still Alice
By Lisa Genova

Surviving Alzheimer's: Practical Tips and Soul-saving Wisdom for Caregivers
By Paula Spencer Scott

The 36-Hour Day: A Family Guide to Caring for People with Alzheimer Disease, Other Dementias, and Memory Loss in Later Life (5th edition)
By Nancy L. Mace, Peter V. Rabins, MD, PhD

The Aftereffects of Caregiving
By Gary Joseph LeBlanc

The Best Friends Approach to Alzheimer's Care
By Virginia Bell, MSW, and David Troxel, MPH

The Best Friends Book of Alzheimer's Activities, Volume One and Two
By Virginia Bell, MSW, David Troxel, MPH, Robin Hamon, MSW, and Tonya Cox, MSW

The Best Friends Staff: Building a Culture of Care in Alzheimer's Programs
By Virginia Bell, MSW, David Troxel, MPH, Robin Hamon, MSW, and Tonya Cox, MSW

The Complete Eldercare Planner: Where to Start, Which Questions to Ask, and How to Find Help (2nd Ed.)
By Joy Loverde

The Validation Breakthrough: Simple Techniques for Communicating with People with Alzheimer's-Type Dementia, Second Edition
By Naomi Feil, MSW

Through the Wilderness of Alzheimer's: A Guide in Two Voices
By Robert and Anne Simpson

Treasure for Alzheimer's: Reflecting on experiences with the art of Lester E. Potts, Jr.
By Richard L. Morgan PhD , Daniel C. Potts MD

Understanding Difficult Behaviors: Some Practical Suggestions for coping with Alzheimer's Disease & Related Illnesses
By Anne Robinson, MA, Beth Spencer, MSW, Laura White, MSW

Validation Techniques for Dementia Care
By Vicki De Klerk-Rubin RN MBA MSW

What's Happening to Grandpa?
By Maria Shriver

While I Still Can
By Rick Phelps and Gary Joseph LeBlanc

Your Brain Health Lifestyle
By Dr. Paul Nussbaum

You Say Goodbye and We Say Hello: The Montessori Method for Positive Dementia Care
By Tom and Karen Brenner

II.

Directory of Organizations and Resources

Alzheimer's Association
225 North Michigan Avenue
Floor 17
Chicago, IL   60601-7633
info@alz.org
http://www.alz.org
Tel: 312-335-8700
1-800-272-3900 (24-hour helpline)

Association for Frontotemporal
Degeneration (AFTD)
Radnor Station Building #2 Suite 320
290 King of Prussia Road
Radnor, PA   19087
info@theaftd.org
http://www.theaftd.org
Tel: 267-514-7221

BrightFocus Foundation
22512 Gateway Center Drive
Clarksburg, MD   20871
info@brightfocus.org
http://www.brightfocus.org/alzheimers/
Tel: 1- 800-437-2423

Department of Veterans Affairs (VA)
Public Affairs & Inter-government
Affairs/Consumer Affairs Service (075B)
810 Vermont Avenue, N.W.
Washington, DC 20420
Tel: 800-827-1000
Email: **consumeraffairs@mail.va.gov**
http://www.va.gov

Family Caregiver Alliance/
National Center on Caregiving
785 Market St.,
Suite 750
San Francisco, CA   94103
info@caregiver.org
http://www.caregiver.org
Tel: 1-800-445-8106

National Family Caregivers Association
10400 Connecticut Avenue
Suite 500
Kensington, MD   20895-3944
info@thefamilycaregiver.org
http://www.thefamilycaregiver.org
Tel: 800-896-3650

National Institute of Mental Health (NIMH)

National Institutes of Health, DHHS
6001 Executive Blvd. Rm. 8184, MSC 9663
Bethesda, MD   20892-9663
http://www.nia.nih.gov/alzheimers
http://www.nimh.nih.gov
Tel: 1-866-415-8051

National Parkinson's Foundation

200 SE 1st Street
Suite 800
Miami, Florida 33131
Toll-free Helpline: 1-800-4PD-INFO
(473-4636)
E-mail inquiries: contact@parkinson.org
www.parkinsons.org

National Respite Network and Resource Center

800 Eastowne Drive
Suite 105
Chapel Hill, NC   27514
http://www.archrespite.org
Tel: 919-490-5577 x222
Fax: 919-490-4905

National Organization for Rare Disorders (NORD)

55 Kenosia Avenue
Danbury, CT   06810
orphan@rarediseases.org
http://www.rarediseases.org
Tel: 203-744-0100
Voice Mail 800-999-NORD (6673)

National Stroke Association

Tel: 1-800-STROKES (787-6537)
9707 E. Easter Lane, Suite B
Centennial, CO 80112
info@stroke.org
http://www.stroke.org/

Project Lifesaver International

201 SW Port St. Lucie Blvd Suite 202
Port St. Lucie, Florida 34984
Tel: 772-446-1271
www.projectlifesaver.org

Social Security Administration

6401 Security Blvd.
Windsor Park Building
Baltimore, MD 21235
Tel: 410-966-3000/800-772-1213
Fax: 410-965-0696
http://www.ssa.gov/reach.htm

9 781478 768760